Azzam scale
in
practical guide of occupational therapy

Ass. Prof. Dr. Ahmed M. Azzam

Department of Physiotherapy for Developmental
Disturbance and
Pediatric Surgery, Faculty of Physical Therapy,
Cairo University

Department of rehabilitation science,
Faculty of applied medical science,
King Saud University
2019

ISBN
978-1-5437-4955-7 (sc)
978-1-5437-4954-0 (e)

Library of Congress Control Number: 2019932552

Print information available on the last page.

To order additional copies of this book, contact
Toll Free 800 101 2657 (Singapore)
Toll Free 1 800 81 7340 (Malaysia)
www.partridgepublishing.com/singapore
orders.singapore@partridgepublishing.com

02/04/2019

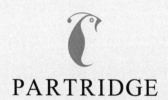

PARTRIDGE

Azzam scale

in

Practical guide of occupational therapy
PART I

Ass. Prof. Dr. Ahmed M. Azzam

Department of Physiotherapy for Developmental Disturbance and Pediatric Surgery, Faculty of Physical Therapy,

Cairo University

Department of rehabilitation science, Faculty of applied medical science, King Saud University

2019

<u>Preface</u>

This book is a compact and accessible guide to the wide range practice of occupational therapy. I feel too much gratitude to our **professor Dr. Emam El negmy** for his deep, continuous guidance, support, advices and consultation from time to time. Also too much gratitude to all our **professors in department** of physiotherapy for growth and development disturbance and pediatric surgery for their support and advices. Fine motor skills problems are discussed as they are presented to the clinician giving background information and guidance. The main aim of this book is evaluating the level of skill should be started with in the treatment program and continuous on that level till be learned enough then changed to more advanced one on the levels of graduations of material used in occupational therapy till the trained skill be acquired. Common underlying mechanisms of skill levels graduations are demonstrated. This book illustrates the underlying principles of skill follow up and re-acquisition of lost skills. This book is divided into 5 main sections. The first is about fine motor skill development and its difference with gross motor skills. Furthermore it gives more light on pyramidal and extra-pyramidal role in fine and gross motor skill control, also more light on the characteristics of upper and lower motor neuron lesion. In section 2 the reader learn the motor learning theory. In section 3 the clinician learns about the graduations level of skill acquisition according to Azzam reacquisition hand skill grading scale to locate the accurate level of skill level suitable for patient dysfunction. In section 4 demonostrate the standardized tests used for evaluation of fine motor skill. Section 5 demonstrated the underlying mechanisms of controlling of spasticity in addition to fine motor skills training (grasping, voluntary release, eye hand co ordination, hand manipulative skills, bilateral hand use and reaching). This book is useful for physical and occupational therapist specially pediatric physical therapists and pediatric occupational therapists.

Ahmed Azzam

Contents

Section 3
Azzam reacquisition hand skill grading scale

Section 4
Evaluation of fine motor skill

Section 5
Treatment of fine motor disorders

Section 6

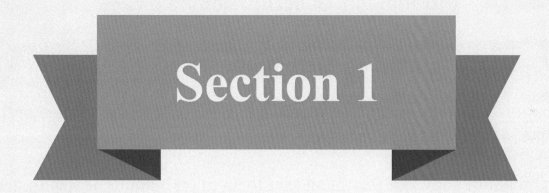

Section 1

Occupational therapy

- Definitions
- kids referred to O.T
- Aims of O.T
- Differences between physical therapy and occupational therapy
- Importance of pyramidal and extra-pyramidal tracts in fine and gross motor skills control
- Occupational therapy present in these areas
- Fine motor skills development
- Neurophysiological characteristics of the hand
- Characteristics of upper and lower motor neuron lesion

Introduction to occupational therapy

Definition:

Occupational therapy is the use of activities as therapeutic tools by remove obstacles or makes them manageable.

Occupational therapy is a treatment that focuses on helping people to achieve independence in all areas of their lives can offer children with various Positive needs and activities to improve their cognitive, physical and motor skills.

Kids referred to OT:

- Cerebral palsy
- Birth injury or birth defects
- Sensory processing/integrative disorders
- Traumatic injuries (brain or spinal cord)
- Learning problem
- Autism
- Developmental disorders
- Juvenile rheumatoid arthritis
- Broken bones or other orthopedic injuries
- Post surgical conditions
- Burns
- Spina bifida
- Cancer
- Sever hand injuries

Aims of occupational therapy:

- Help kids with sever developmental delay to learn some basic tasks as bathing, dressing, brushing their teeth, feeding themselves.
- Help kids with behavioral disorders to learn anger management techniques (Instead of hitting others learn positive ways to deal with anger as writing about feelings or participating in physical activities).

- Teach kids with physical disabilities the coordination skills required to feed themselves, use computer, increase speed of hand writing.
- Evaluate each child needs for specialized equipment, dressing devices, communication aids.
- Work with kids who have sensory and attentional disorders to improve focus and social skills.

Difference between physical therapy and occupational therapy:

Physical therapy deals with pain, strength, joint range of motion, endurance and gross motor functioning. Whereas occupational therapy deals more with fine motor skills, visual-perceptual skills, cognitive skills and sensory-processing deficits.

Table 1) Importance of pyramidal and extra-pyramidal tracts in fine and gross motor skills control:

Pyramidal T	Extrapyramidal T
1-only one neuron from cortex to A.H.Cs without synapse	1-multiple neurons from cortex to AHCs with many synapse
2-occupies pyramid of medulla	2-don't occupy the pyramid
3-origin localized(area 4) and area 8	3-origin wide (all cortical areas with area 6 on top)
4-85% of fibers cross to opposite side at pyramide 15% cross at cervical level	4-some tracts cross and others don't
5-doesnot function in first year of life(not yet mylinated)i.e. undeveloped	5-function in first year of life
6-facilitatory to muscle tone and deep reflexes (pure lesion decrease tone and reflexes). pure lesion occur at area 4 only	6-some tracts are facilitatory but others inhibitory. Lesion lead to increase tone and reflexes

7- responsible for fine isolated and skillful movements as in hand function(grasping, voluntary release, eye hand co ordination, hand manipulative skills, bilateral hand use, reaching) It initiates voluntary movements	7-responsible for gross movement using large groups of muscles As (sitting skills, swinging arm during walking) They coordinate voluntary movements

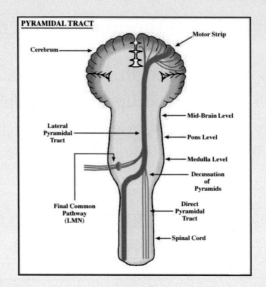

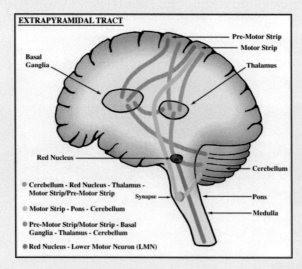

Fig (1): pyramidal and extra-pyramidal tracts

<u>Occupational therapy present in these areas:</u>

- Hospitals
- Schools
- Rehabilitation centers
- Mental health facilities
- Private practices
- Children clinic
- Nursing home

<u>Fine Motor Development (FMD)</u>
<u>Development of hand functioning:</u>

0-3months:
Assumes fisted hand

3-5months:
Bring hands together in midline
Clumsy reaching attempts
Grasp object placed in hand

5-7 months:
Reaching successfully in all directions
Bilateral reach become unilateral reach by7 months
Ulnar grasp changing to palmer grasp
Mouthing

7-9 months:
Transfer objects from hand to hand
Unilateral reach, grasp
Holds one block while given another
Offer cube but cannot release it

9-12 months:
Grasp with trunk rotation

Pokes objects with finger

Grasps between fingers and thumb then one finger and thumb

Reach and grasp possible in all direction

more precise release until places small objects in jar

12-15 months:

Build tower of two cubes

Pushes pulls large toys

Drink alone from cup

15 months to 2years:

Delicate pincer grasp

Takes off shoes

Turn pages of book

Strings large beads later small beads

Scribbles with pencil

2 years:

Increase fine movement

Throw ball accurately

Screws, unscrew lids, toys

3 years:

Take off all clothes

Feeds self completely

Copies circle

Cuts with scissor

Wash alone

4 years:

Draw simple house

Brush teeth

Constructive building include 3 steps with cubes

Matches, names four colour

5 years:
Copies square, triangle, letters
Matches 12 colours
Use knife, fork
Dressed, undressed completely

The arm and hand are subject to more complex neuronal control. Before initiating a purposeful motor act such as grasping an object, the nervous system needs information. Vision describes the shape of the object, its location, and its distance from the body. Proprioceptive input defines the condition of the inner world and the position of the limbs and trunk. The brain searches for stored memories of similar situations. Once the object is touched, cutaneous Proprioceptive sensation updates the recorded memories of weight, surface, and shape.

The neuro- physiological characteristics of the hand include:

1. Had greater number of muscle spindle and GTO which provide hand with great control
2. Great representation in sensory area via great number of tactile receptors
3. Broad tips of finger to increase exposed area for distinguishing between materials
4. Presence of the web space between thumb and index provide freely movement of thumb to occupy 50% hand function
5. Purely supplied by 15-20% of directly pyramidal tracts on alpha, gamma motor neuron

Diminished afferent input to the brain from the affected hand is a common deficit after stroke. Patients become less aware of their affected upper extremity because of sensory loss and partial paralysis. As a consequence, they use that extremity less and less, learning to use the unaffected arm in its place. Over time, disuse weakens muscles and most likely reduces the representation area of the affected part in the cortex

Table 2) Characteristics of upper and lower motor neuron lesion:

Characteristics of UMNL-LMNL	Upper motor neuron lesion	Lower motor neuron lesion
1-Paralysis - extend - side - type - recovery	- wide spread - opposite side - spastic - no recovery theoretically But recovery occur under umbrella of neural plasticity	- localized - same side - flaccid - complete recovery in neuro-praxia Incomplete recovery in axonotemeses No-recovery of neurotemeses
2-muscle tone	Hypertonia (spastic, Rigidity, fluctuating hypertonia) Inhibitory tracts from cortex and corpus striatum are damaged but facilitatory vestibule-spinal and reticulo-spinal are working	Hypotonia (mild, moderate,flaccidity) Due to reflex arch is damaged
3-reflexes - superficial reflexes	- lost as abdominal reflex - positive response as babinski sign extension big toe due to pyramidal tract lesion+ fanning of other toes due to extra pyramidal tract lesion	- lost as abdominal reflex - In partial lesion negative response (flexion of all toes occur) - In complete lesion lost of response occur
- deep reflexes	- hyper-reflexia	- hypo-reflexia

4-wasting of muscle	- no wasting except with neglection(disuse atrophy)	- marked atrophy occur due to reflex arch is interrupted lead to loss of pumping action of muscle lead to protein catabolism inside muscle (sarcomere) decrease the muscle contour
5-response to electric stimulation	- normal response to electric stimulation(negative response)	- reaction of degeneration (positive response) occur in LMNL due to complete cut of reflex arch(in ability to respond to electrical stimulation) - normal esponse(negative response) occur in partial lesion
6-blood supply - **metabolism**	- normal response	- decreased due to interruption of reflex arch

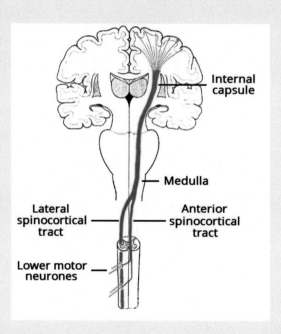

Fig (2): upper and lower motor neuron

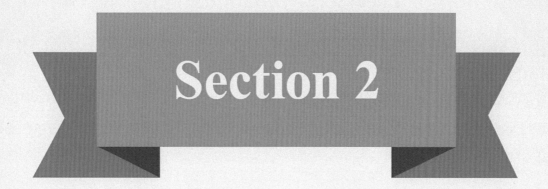

Motor learning

- Theories in rehabilitation
- Motor learning process
- Forms of learning
- Underlying mechanism of hand function training
- Underlying mechanism of skill acquisition
- Learning and memory
- Feed back
- Practice conditions
- Recovery of function
- Neural plasticity
- Sensory perceptual system

Theories in rehabilitation

There are three main theories in pediatric rehabilitations:

1-Neuro-Developmental Theory.

2-Sensory-Motor integration Theory.

3-Motor Learning Theory (closed-loop theory-schema theory-dynamics systems theory).

In occupational therapy practice the dominant theoretical approaches used are sensory integration (S.I) approach and neuro-developmental (N.D) approach these approaches were developed in 1960s and 1940s respectively are based on hierarchical model of CNS since the late of 1980s the CNS has been conceptualized as multilevel and multisystem rather than hierarchical this shift in thinking about the CNS lead to development of contemporary theories of motor learning

Motor learning process

Definition of terms

Perception:

Is the integration of sensory impression into psychologically meaningful information progressing through various processing stages each stage is controlled by specific brain structures that process sensory information at different levels from initial stage of sensory to increasingly abstract levels of interpretation and integration in higher levels of the brain .Higher center integrate inputs from many senses and interpretate incoming sensory information then form motor plan and strategies for action thus a higher levels may select the specific response to accomplish a particular task.

Cognition

Is the ability to process, sort, retrieve and manipulate information.

Include attention motivation and emotional aspects of motor control.

Motor control

is the ability to regulate the mechanisms essentials to movement include perception and cognition(action system that are organized to achieve specific goals)

Functional skills

1-Bed mobility tasks (moving from supine to sit, to the edge of bed and back,change position within bed)

2-Transfer tasks(moving from sitting to stand and back, moving on to and off a toilet)

3-Activity of daily living (dressing, toileting, grooming and feeding)

Task

According to whether the base of support is still or in motion task is divided into stability and mobility.

Stability tasks such as sitting or standing are performed with anon moving base of support

Mobility tasks such as walking and running is a moving base of support

In between them are tasks has more complex movement over a modified base of support as moving from sitting to standing

Learning: process of acquiring knowledge about the world

Motor learning: set of processes associated with practice or experience leading to relatively permanent changes in the capability for producing skilled action

Motor learning concepts:

Learning is a process of acquiring the capability for skilled action

Learning result from experience or practice

Learning cannot be measured directly instead it is inferred from behavior

Learning produce relatively permanent changes in behavior

Motor learning involve more than motor processes .it involve learning new strategies for sensing as well as moving .thus motor learning like motor control emerge from a complex of perception –cognition action processes

Changes in performance that resulted from practice were usually thought to reflect changes in learning thus learning produce relatively permanent change but performance produce a temporary change in motor behavior seen during practice sessions or transfer tasks

Forms of learning:

1-Non associative learning:

A-Habituation: a decrease in response that occurs as a result of repeated exposure to non painful stimuli.
Used in treatment of dizzy in patients with vestibular dysfunction.
Patients are asked to move repeatedly in way that provoke their dizznya this repetition result in habituation to dizziness response

B-Sensitization: increased responsiveness following noxious stimulus.
Used in balance training as the child when fall during walking in the second time he thought about his fallen so he maintain his balance

2-Associated learning:

A-Classical condition: learning to pair two stimuli during classical condition an initially weak stimulus (the conditioned stimulus or CS) become highly effective in producing a response when it becomes associated with another stronger stimulus (un conditioned stimulus)
- Before learning
CS.lead to no response
UCS lead to UCR
- After learning
CS lead to CR (formerly called UCR)
thus as patients gain skills we see then move along the continuum of assistance from hands on assistance from the therapist to performing the task with verbal cues and eventually to performing the action un assisted.

B-Operant condition: trials and error learning behavior that are rewarded tend to be repeated at the cost of other behavior

3-Procedure and Declarative learning

A-Procedural learning:

during motor skills acquisition,repeating a movement continually under varying circumstances typically leads to procedural learning and automatically learn the movement itself e.g. patients learn to move from chair of different heights and at different position relative to the bed this learning enable them to transfer safely in un familiar circumstances

B-Declarative learning: depend on knowledge that can be consciously recalled thus require awareness attention e.g., patient said i button the top button then the next one so constant repetition can transform declarative into procedural knowledge

Learning and memory

May be seen as a continuum from short term change in the efficiency or strength of synaptic connections to long term structural changes in the organization and numbers of connections among neurons

Learning can be seen as a continuum of short term to long term changes in the ability to produce skilled action

Practice lead to increase of synaptic efficiency lead to gradually developed structural changes (long term modification of behavior)

Neural modifiability:

Change in synaptic efficiency lead to change in synaptic connection through persistence change

Continuum learning:

Short term changes lead to long term changes through persistence change

Like learning is the recovery of function characterized by a continuum changes immediately follow injury like unmasking of existence to long term structural changes such as remapping of sensory or motor cortex

Learning is defined as the acquisition of knowledge or ability

Memory is the retention and storage of that knowledge or ability

Memory storage divided into

1-Short term memory:
Refer to working memory which has a limited capacity of information and lasts for a few moments. It reflect a momentary attention to something such as when we remember a phone number only long enough to dial it then it is gone

2-Long term memory:
Related to the process of learning .Initial stage of long term memory formation reflect functional change in the efficiency of synapses. later stage of memory reflect structural changes in synaptic connections

Loss of memory abilities was not related to site of lesion but to the extend of lesion of the cortex

Learning alters our capability for acting by changing both the effectiveness and anatomic connections of neural pathways

Feed back

Definition:
Broadest definition include all of the sensory information that is available as the result of a movement

Types:

Intrinsic feedback:
Is a feed back that comes to the individual simply through various sensory systems as a result of the normal production of movement This include visual information, somato sensory information concerning the position of the limbs as one was moving.

2-Extrinsic feedback:
Is the information that supplement intrinsic feedback For ex. When you tell a patient that he need to step higher to clear an object while walking you are offering extrinsic feedback.

3-Terminal feedback:

Occur when extrinsic feedback given concurrently with the task and at the end of the task e.g. Verbal or manual guidance to the hand of the patient learning him to reach for object .Telling the patients who has made a first unsuccessful attempt to rise from a chair that he should push harder the next time using the arms to create more force to stand up.

Practice conditions:

The more practice lead to more sensory input lead to more feedback lead to permanent changes as new strategies and motor plan produced lead to learning a new skill or restore the lost skill.

Types of practice:

1-Massed practice:

Session in which the amount of practice time is greater than the amount of rest between trials.

2-Distributed practice:

Session in which the amount of rest between trials equals or is greater than the amount of time for a trial

Recovery of function

Definition:

Is the reacquisition of movement skills lost through injury, achieving function through original process

Motor learning:

Is the study of the acquisition or modification of movement skill.

Compensation:

Is an achieving function through alternative process which lead to alternative behavioral strategies are adapted to complete a task. The function return but not in its identical premorbid form

Factors affecting recovery of function:

1-Effect of age:
Injury during infancy cause a fewer deficits than damage in the adult period Damage to the dominant hemisphere show little or no effect on speech in infants but causes varying degrees of aphasia in adults .it explain that the brain react differently to injury at different stages of development.

2-Characteristics of lesion:
A-Small lesion has a greater chance of recovery as long as no functional area has been removed
B-Slowly developing lesion cause less functional loss than lesions that happen quickly
C-Function is spared if a similar lesion is made serially over time

3-Effect of experience (environmental effect):
Enriched subjects may have developed functional neural circuit that is more varied than that of restricted subjects. This provide them with greater ability to reorganize the nervous system after a lesion or simply to use alternative pathways to perform a task. To affect recovery of function environmental stimulation must incorporate active participation of the patient for full recovery to occur.

4-Effect of training:
When training was delayed recovery was worse than when it was started immediately following the lesion .brain injury must be treated as soon after the damage has occur to ensure maximum effectiveness.

levels control perception and movement:
Information coming from periphery (muscles, joint, skin) and from skin, muscles of the head,vestibular system, vision to brain stem then to cerebral cortex lead

to making a plane or strategies then theses signals go to cerebellum and basal ganglion which modify it,refine the movement then cerebellum send update of the movement output plans to motor cortex again sending descending signals to activate final common pathway(motor neuron) which activate the muscles to gain reaching grasping and eye hand co ordination.

Higher brain center integrate input from many senses and interpretate incoming sensory information then form motor plan and strategies for action thus a higher levels may select the specific response to accomplish a particular task

Neural plasticity:

We know that the nervous system develops by making new connections between neurons throughout life. As some connections disappear through disuse, other connections can be formed as a result of new experience. So the brain is able to make adaptations at any age.

1-Denervation super- sensitivity:
Denervation of part of organs stimulate the healthy part to increase its efficiency to compensate the lost function of degenerated part.

2-Resolution of edema:
Efficiency of venous system and villi is responsible for decreasing of central edema gradually this illustrate the gradual improvement of patients.

3-Diachasis:
The neighbor cells of degenerated cells are shocked (no organic lesion) loss its function temporary and after finishing of the shock stage this neighbor cells will recovered and this explore the improvement after the shock stage.

4-Axonal sprouting:
Motor neuron is regenerated by sprouting from 1-4 mm every day.

5-Collateral sprouting:

Alternating routes occur to reach the healthy dendrites by healthy axon to exclude the dead cell. This will illustrate the regaining of function after long time of training.

6-Unmasking of silent synapse:

Brain contain more than 33 trillion cell .Not all of them are actively participated in brain functions. The function is occupied by competition in two ways either new skill gained by long run training forming new neuronal circuit.

Other route of activation of silent synapses occur after lesion and dead of some cells so silent synapses become active and uncovering of the silent synapses occur and the functions of the dead cell transferred to the new active synapses and new skill gained by long run training forming new neuronal circuit.

Sensory perceptual system

Sensory inputs serve as the stimuli for reflexive movement .sensory information has a vital role in modulating output of movement

Peripheral receptors

1-Muscle spindle:

They consists of intra-fusal muscle fiber-muscle spindle increased in anti gravity muscles,concentrate in extra ocular, hand and neck muscle as we use theses muscles in eye head and eye hand co ordination, grasping and reaching for objects and move about in the environment.

2-joint receptor:
- Ruffini type ending
- Spray ending
- Pacinian corpuscle
- Ligament receptor
- Free nerve ending

Afferent information from peripheral receptors ascend to cerebral cortex contribute to our perception of position in space so CNS determine joint position by monitoring which receptors are activated at the same time this allow for determination of exact joint position.

3-Cutaneous receptor:
Mechano receptors as pacinian, merkles, misners, ruffini, hair follicle
Thermo receptors: sensed to temperature change
Nociceptors: as pain receptors

4-vestibular receptors:
Transport two types of information; the position of head in space and sudden change in direction of movement of the head.

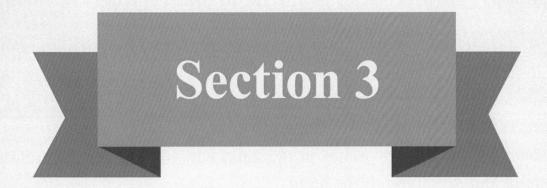

Section 3

Azzam reacquisition hand skill grading scale

- Anatomical characteristics of the hand and relations of the hand
- Indications of Azzam reacquisition hand skill grading scale
- Graduations used to follow the improvement in Azzam reacquisition hand skill grading scale In rehabilitation
- Eight evaluative parameters determine the characteristics of materials used for evaluation and treatment by Azzam reacquisition hand skill grading scale
- The size, shape, weight, texture, and slipperiness of the objects must be given careful consideration in Azzam reacquisition hand skill grading scale
- Time, speed, accuracy and numbers of trials they are movement parameters have to be evaluated in Azzam reacquisition hand skill grading scale
- Guidelines scoring of subtests of Azzam reacquisition hand skill grading scale
- Azzam subtests hand skill levels of progression
- The underlying mechanism of Azzam reacquisition hand skill grading scale
- APPENDIX
- Material used in Azzam reacquisition hand skill grading scale

Anatomical characteristics of the hand and relations of the hand:

1-The most important physical movement related to hand function is supination due to it allow free thumb movement

2-Thumb act as a leader for the hand function. Thumb represent 50% of hand function, index 20% and other 3 fingers 30%

3- Presence of Mechanical arches in the hand which allow for different types of grasping and reshaping of the hand

4- Presence of web space allow free movement of the thumb and performing delicate grasp

5- Broad tips of finger to increase exposed area for distinguishing between materials

Neurophysiological characteristics of the hand:

1-All hand functions (grasping-voluntary release-eye hand coordination-bilateral hand use and grasping phase of reaching) depend mainly on pyramidal control except transport phase of reaching depend mainly on extra-pyramidal control.

2-Had greater number of muscle spindle and GTO which provide hand with great control.

3-Great mapping representation in sensory area via great number of tactile receptors.

4 -Purely supplied by 15-20% of directly pyramidal tracts on alpha, gamma motor neuron of hand muscles stretch reflex.

5-Highly innervated hand muscles motor units .It contain great nerve supply with less muscle fibers.

Indications of Azzam reacquisition hand skill grading scale in rehabilitation:

1-Delayed hand functions in C.P.

2-In erbs palsy when C7 involved the wrist is dropped with ulnar deviation

3-In klumpkes paralysis as a result of lesion of C8,T1

4-Fisted hand as in hemiplegic cerebral palsy

5-Involuntary hand movement (stereo typed) as in dyskinesia

6-Incoordinated hand as in ataxia

7-Pronated hand due tightness of pronator as in hemiplegia and erbs palsy

8-Traumatic hand limitations post plaster cast

9- Post –operative hand limitations (intramedullary nails,plate and screw,tendon transfer and soft tissue release)

10- Congenital hand as in arthrogryposis

11-Shorted hand and upper limb

12-Painful hand as in juvenile rheumatoid arthritis

13-Ape hand

14-Claw hand

15-Drop wrist

16-Hand disorders as dupuetren contracture and trigger finger

Azzam reacquisition hand skill grading scale

It consists of 42 subtests according to 8 parameters including : **-Object characteristics (size, shape, weight, and texture of material): Size:** small-big **Shape:** rectangular-square-circular **Weight:** heavy-light **Texture of material:** rough- smooth.

- Plus factors affecting on performance (reaction time, speed, accuracy, and numbers of trials). Time: elevated or diminished **Speed:** elevated or diminished **Accuracy:** elevated or diminished **Numbers of trials:** elevated or diminished .

- Guidelines scoring of subtests: table (3) We start evaluation by detecting the intention level of hand skill progression in all tests. The scale consists of 42 subtests of hand skill levels progression Each subtest is scored by the examiner on a scale from I to v points according to the guidelines for scoring. Rating scale grade from I (complete loss of hand skills) to II(Poorly developed skill) to Ш(Acceptable developed skill) to Iv (Nearly developed skill) to v (complete re-acquisition of hand skills) A cut-off score of 21 suggests a partial loss of hand skills(grade Ш of skill). The score was calculated by detecting the level of progression could be reached.

-Azzam subtests hand skill levels of progression: table (4) Using Azzam reacquisition skill grading scale by manipulating the object characteristics according to 8 parameters and 42 subtests levels of progressions this lead to the dedication of the progression level of hand dexterity. Started with(1-Big object, rectangular shape, rough, heavy, ↑time, ↓speed, ↑accuracy, ↓numbers of trials) and the last and more difficult one is(42-Small object, circular, smooth, light, ↓time, ↑speed, ↓accuracy, ↑number of trials) It was performed before starting the therapy and after 12 weeks of it.

Graduations used to follow the improvement in Azzam reacquisition hand skill grading scale

These graduations used to evaluate and follow up the improvement of all fine motor skills to locate the grade and characteristics of materials used for both evaluation and treatment.

We use these graduations to determine the level of skill recovered as evaluation for all hand functions skills (grasping, voluntary release,eye hand co ordination, hand manipulative skills, bilateral hand use and reaching) . After determine the level of skill as grade number (1,2,3……..) this grade become the main training till we end from this grade and change to more advanced grade till we reach the nearly normal skill performance.

All hand functions skills evaluated and treated under the umbrella of these characteristics of material used in O.T

Eight evaluative parameters determine the characteristics of materials used for evaluation and treatment by Azzam reacquisition hand skill grading scale:

1-Size:
One important parameter used in evaluation first graduations used big size of the material because it is more easy for hand functions(grasping-voluntary

release-eye hand co ordination-hand manipulative skills-bilateral hand use-reaching) in more difficult graduations we used the smaller size material materials as beads because the more smaller of the material the more difficult in grasping and other fine motor skills .

2-**Shape**:

Another important parameter used in evaluation first graduations used rectangular or triangular shapes of material .It is more easy because they have more edges and different surfaces. In more difficult graduations we use circular materials because they haven't edges and contain one surface so it is more difficult in grasping and other fine motor skills.

3-**Weight**:

Another important parameter used in evaluation first graduations used the heavy material because it is more easy due to it is more stable. In more difficult graduations we use light materials because it is less stable so it is more difficult in grasping and other fine motor skills.

4- **Texture and Slipperiness:**

Another important parameter used in evaluation first graduations used the rough material because it is more easy due to they increase friction force with the hand In more difficult graduations we use a smooth materials because it is less friction force with hand so it is more difficult in grasping and other fine motor skills.

5-**Reaction time:**

Another important parameter used in evaluation first graduations we increase the reaction time because it is more easy due to this will decrease the speed of performance and increase the accuracy and decrease of number of trials

Reaction time=distance/speed

Reaction time α accuracy

Reaction time α 1/number of trials

In more difficult graduations we use less reaction time because it is more difficult in grasping and other fine motor skills.

6-Speed:

Another important parameter used in evaluation first graduations we decrease the speed of performance because it is easier due to this will increase the reaction time of performance and increase the accuracy and decrease of number of trials.

Speed=distance/ reaction time

Speed α 1/ accuracy

Speed α number of trials

In more difficult graduations we use more speed performance because it is more difficult in grasping and other fine motor skills.

7-Accuracy:

Another important parameter used in evaluation first graduations we increase the accuracy of performance because it is more easy due to this will be increased with increased reaction time and be decreased with increased of speed and decrease of number of trials.

Accuracy α reaction time

Accuracy α 1/number of trials

Accuracy α1/speed

In more difficult graduations we use less accuracy because it is more difficult in grasping and other fine motor skills.

8-Number of trials:

Another important parameter used in evaluation first graduations it will be decreased with increased reaction time and be increased with increased of speed and decrease of accuracy.

Number of trials α speed

Number of trials α 1/accuracy

Number of trials α 1/reaction time

The size, shape, weight, texture, and slipperiness of the objects must be given careful consideration in Azzam reacquisition hand skill grading scale

Children can handle blocks and other objects with straight sides more effectively than round objects .Grasp of small tiny object should not be the priority for children,people use an opposed pattern to grasp items as a cup(cylindrical grasp,a ball (aspheric grasp),a telephone receiver and a large block Children with disability be assisted in developing skills of all types of opposed grasp pattern,power grasp,and lateral pinch.

Time, speed, accuracy and numbers of trials they are movement parameters have to be evaluated in Azzam reacquisition hand skill grading scale

To be able to gain skill we have to bring hands to the right place at the right time as catching a ball to catch the ball successfully the hand has to be at the calculated meeting point at exactly the right time. In a reaching movement the goal is to transport the hand to the target with precision in both time and space, it also refers to the path taken by the hand as it moves toward a target and the speed as it moves along the path

Timing places high demands on the motor system for speed and efficiency with high demands for attention and perception.

Reaction time provides an indication of an individual speed in preparing a response.

Production of fast arm movement to achieve a goal may be affected by poor attention as clumsy children A small object require longer reaching time than larger object the first part of the movement seems to be unaffected by object size but for smaller objects extra movement time is spent in the last part of movement when we increase the speed of a movement the accuracy will decrease

Table 3) Guidelines scoring of subtests of Azzam reacquisition hand skill grading scale

Skill grade	Description	Characteristics	Initial assessment	Levels training
I	Lost skill	Can not perform the first level of skill progression	For locating the skill level of progression Then by re-evaluation for locating the new level	Gaining of the specific level of progression obtained by massed practice at that level
II	Poorly developed skill	Can perform less than 10th levels of progression		
III	Acceptable developed skill	Can perform less than 20th levels of progression		
Iv	Nearly developed skill	Can perform all levels of progression except the last one		
v	Well developed skill	Can perform all levels perfectly		

Table 4) Azzam subtests hand skill levels of progression

1-Big object, rectangular shape, rough, heavy, ↑time, ↓speed, ↑accuracy, ↓numbers of trials

2-Big object, rectangular shape, rough, heavy, ↓time, ↑speed, ↓accuracy, ↑number of trials

3-Big object, square shape, rough, heavy, ↑time, ↓speed, ↑accuracy, ↓numbers of trials

4-Big object, square shape, rough, heavy, ↓time, ↑speed, ↓accuracy, ↑number of trials

5-Big object, rectangular, rough, light, ↑time, ↓speed, ↑accuracy, ↓numbers of trials

6-Big object, rectangular, rough, light, ↓time, ↑speed, ↓accuracy, ↑number of trials

7-Big object, rectangular, smooth, heavy, ↑time, ↓speed, ↑accuracy, ↓numbers of trials

8-Big object, rectangular, smooth, heavy, ↓time, ↑speed, ↓accuracy, ↑number of trials

9-Big object, circular, rough, heavy, ↑time, ↓speed, ↑accuracy, ↓numbers of trials

10-Big object, circular, rough, heavy, ↓time, ↑speed, ↓accuracy, ↑number of trials

11-Big object, rectangular, smooth, light, ↑time, ↓speed, ↑accuracy, ↓numbers of trials

12-Big object, rectangular, smooth, light, ↓time, ↑speed, ↓accuracy, ↑number of trials

13-Big object, circular, smooth, heavy, ↑time, ↓speed, ↑accuracy, ↓numbers of trials

14-Big object, circular, smooth, heavy, ↓time, ↑speed, ↓accuracy, ↑number of trials

15-Big object, circular, smooth, light, ↑time, ↓speed, ↑accuracy, ↓numbers of trials

16-Big object, circular, smooth, light, ↓time, ↑speed, ↓accuracy, ↑number of trials

17-Big object, rectangular, rough, light ↑time, ↓speed, ↑accuracy, ↓numbers of trials

18-Big object, rectangular, rough, light, ↓time, ↑speed, ↓accuracy, ↑number of trials

19-Big object, square, rough, light ↑time, ↓speed, ↑accuracy, ↓numbers of trials

20-Big object, square, rough, light, ↓time, ↑speed, ↓accuracy, ↑number of trials

21-Small object, rectangular, rough, heavy, ↑time, ↓speed, ↑accuracy, ↓numbers of trials

22-Small object, rectangular, rough, heavy, ↓time, ↑speed, ↓accuracy, ↑number of trials

23-Small object, square, rough, heavy, ↑time, ↓speed, ↑accuracy, ↓numbers of trials

24-Small object, square, rough, heavy, ↓time, ↑speed, ↓accuracy, ↑number of trials

25-Small object, circular, rough, heavy, ↑time, ↓speed, ↑accuracy, ↓numbers of trials

26-Small object, circular, rough, heavy, ↓time, ↑speed, ↓accuracy, ↑number of trials

27-Small object, rectangular, smooth, heavy, ↑time, ↓speed, ↑accuracy, ↓numbers of trials

28-Small object, rectangular, smooth, heavy, ↓time, ↑speed, ↓accuracy, ↑number of trials

29-Small object, rectangular, rough, light ↑time, ↓speed, ↑accuracy, ↓numbers of trials

30-Small object, rectangular, rough, light, ↓time, ↑speed, ↓accuracy, ↑number of trials

31-Small object, square, rough, light ↑time, ↓speed, ↑accuracy, ↓numbers of trials

32-Small object, square, rough, light, ↓time, ↑speed, ↓accuracy, ↑number of trials

33-Small object, rectangular, smooth, light, ↑time, ↓speed, ↑accuracy, ↓numbers of trials

34-Small object, rectangular, smooth, light, ↓time, ↑speed, ↓accuracy, ↑number of trials

35-Small object, square, smooth, light, ↑time, ↓speed, ↑accuracy, ↓numbers of trials

36-Small object, square, smooth, light, ↓time, ↑speed, ↓accuracy, ↑number of trials

37-Small object, circular, smooth, heavy, ↑time, ↓speed, ↑accuracy, ↓numbers of trials

38-Small object, circular, smooth, heavy, ↓time, ↑speed, ↓accuracy, ↑number of trials

39-Small object, circular, rough, light, ↑time, ↓speed, ↑accuracy, ↓numbers of trials

40-Small object, circular, rough, light, ↓time, ↑speed, ↓accuracy, ↑number of trials

41-Small object, circular, smooth, light ↑time, ↓speed, ↑accuracy, ↓numbers of trials

42-Small object, circular, smooth, light, ↓time, ↑speed, ↓accuracy, ↑number of trials

<u>The underlying mechanism of Azzam reacquisition hand skill grading scale:</u>

The more practice and repetition are key components of training which lead to more sensory input, feedback and permanent changes as new strategies and motor plan produced lead to learning a new skill or restore the lost skill.

The nervous system provide the:

1-Sensory processing: for perception of body orientation in space provided by visual, vestibular, and somato-sensory systems.

2-Sensory-motor integration: essential for linking sensation to motor responses (centrally programmed postural adjustments that precede voluntary movement).

3-Mechanism of new motor strategy:

Information coming from periphery reached to the spinal cord through spinal nerves, information coming from head and neck reached to brainstem through cranial nerves. All the previous information reached to the thalamus to be sensitized then to the post-central gyrus to be localized. Perception, cognition, new sensory strategy will be produced by sensory areas which lead to increase of efficiency of synapses.

After that information reach to cerebellum and basal ganglion to be smoothening and prevention of excessive activity, then reach to pre-central gyrus to produce permanent changes and new motor behavior.

Which mean learning of new skill then formation of motor command via tracts to final common pathway (alpha and gamma MN) to perform new behavior of skills or reacquisition of skill. Despite the development of indices designed to assess the function of the hand's grip strength assessment remains the cornerstone of most longitudinal studies designed to show functional change in the hand.

Neuro-physiological evidence that cortical reorganization may ensue as a consequence of prolonged sensory input as consequence motor representation areas for evoking a wrist extension movement receive coetaneous input from wide receptive fields located over the volar aspect of the fingers. The evidence for cortical plasticity, in the presence of such functional organization, may provide some insight into the neuro-physiological basis for improved hand motor control.

Fig 3) The underlying mechanism of Azzam hand skills progression scales:

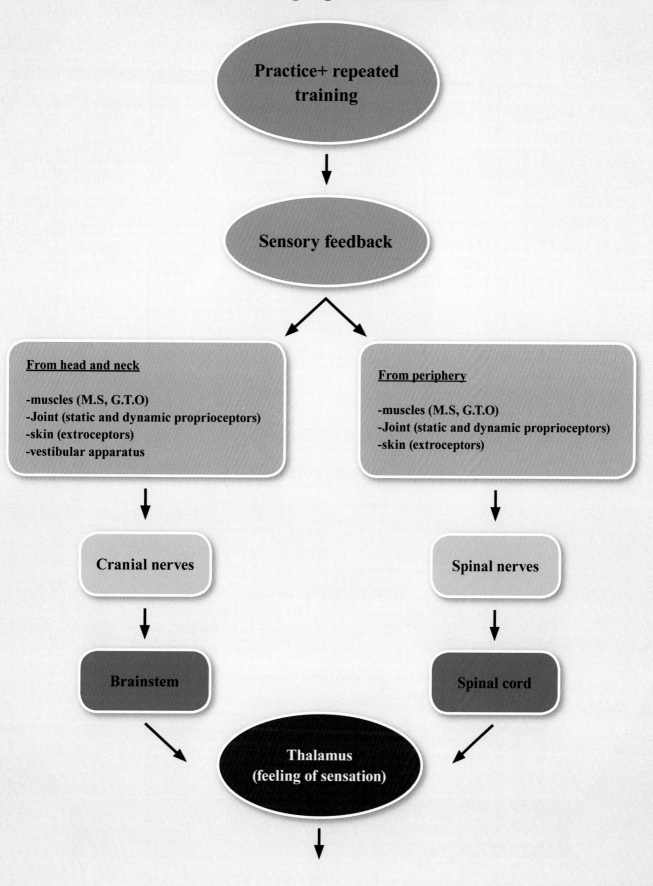

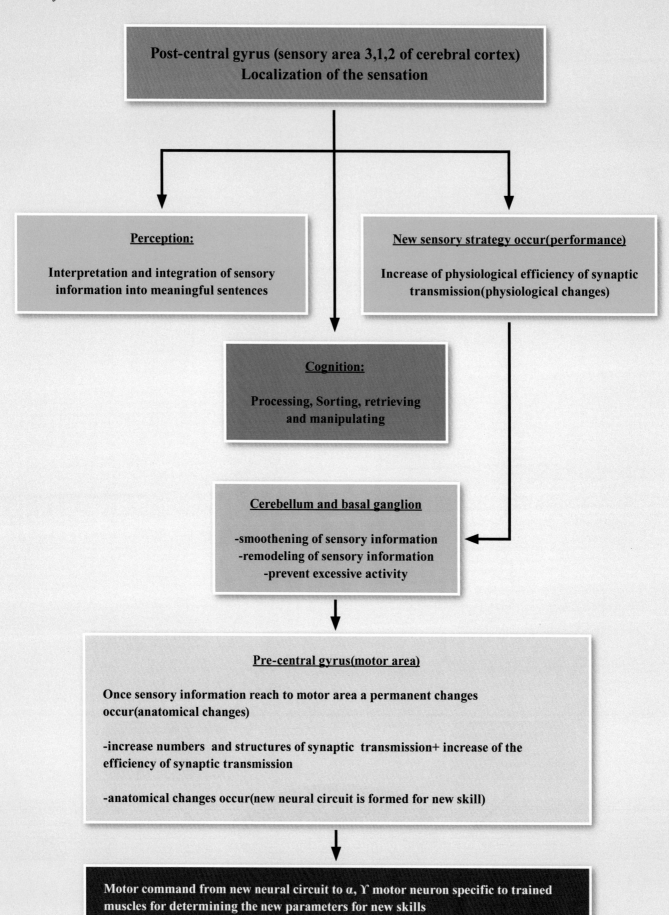

Post-central gyrus (sensory area 3,1,2 of cerebral cortex)
Localization of the sensation

Perception:

Interpretation and integration of sensory information into meaningful sentences

New sensory strategy occur(performance)

Increase of physiological efficiency of synaptic transmission(physiological changes)

Cognition:

Processing, Sorting, retrieving and manipulating

Cerebellum and basal ganglion

-smoothening of sensory information
-remodeling of sensory information
-prevent excessive activity

Pre-central gyrus(motor area)

Once sensory information reach to motor area a permanent changes occur(anatomical changes)

-increase numbers and structures of synaptic transmission+ increase of the efficiency of synaptic transmission

-anatomical changes occur(new neural circuit is formed for new skill)

Motor command from new neural circuit to α, ɣ motor neuron specific to trained muscles for determining the new parameters for new skills

APPENDIX

Table 5) Azzam reacquisition hand skill grading scale

Skill grade	Description	Characteristics	Levels of progression	Initial assessment	Levels training
I	Lost skill	Cannot perform the first level of skill progression	1-Big object, rectangular shape, rough, heavy, ↑time, ↓speed, ↑accuracy, ↓numbers of trials	For locating the skill level of progression Then by re-evaluation for locating the new level	Gaining of the specific level of progression obtained by massed practice at that level
II	Poorly developed skill	Can perform less than 10th levels of progression	2-Big object, rectangular shape, rough, heavy, ↓time, ↑speed, ↓accuracy, ↑number of trials	4-Big object, square shape, rough, heavy, ↓time, ↑speed, ↓accuracy, ↑number of trials	
III	Acceptable developed skill	Can perform less than 20th levels of progression	3-Big object, square shape, rough, heavy, ↑time, ↓speed, ↑accuracy, ↓numbers of trials	5-Big object, rectangular, rough, light, ↑time, ↓speed, ↑accuracy, ↓numbers of trials	
Iv	Nearly developed skill	Can perform all levels of progression except the last one		7- Big object, rectangular, smooth, heavy, ↑time, ↓speed, ↑accuracy, ↓numbers of trials	
v	Well developed skill	Can perform all levels perfectly	6-Big object, rectangular, rough, light, ↓time, ↑speed, ↓accuracy, ↑number of trials	9-Big object, circular, rough, heavy, ↑time, ↓speed, ↑accuracy, ↓numbers of trials	
				11-Big object, rectangular, smooth, light, ↑time, ↓speed, ↑accuracy, ↓numbers of trials	
			8-Big object, rectangular, smooth, heavy, ↓time, ↑speed, ↓accuracy, ↑number of trials	12-Big object, rectangular, smooth, light, ↓time, ↑speed, ↓accuracy, ↑number of trials	
			10-Big object, circular, rough, heavy, ↓time, ↑speed, ↓accuracy, ↑number of trials	13-Big object, circular, smooth, heavy, ↑time, ↓speed, ↑accuracy, ↓numbers of trials	
				15-Big object, circular, smooth, light, ↑time, ↓speed, ↑accuracy, ↓numbers of trials	
			14-Big object, circular, smooth, heavy, ↓time, ↑speed, ↓accuracy, ↑number of trials	16-Big object, circular, smooth, light, ↓time, ↑speed, ↓accuracy, ↑number of trials	
			17-Big object, rectangular, rough, light ↑time, ↓speed, ↑accuracy, ↓numbers of trials	18-Big object, rectangular, rough, light, ↓time, ↑speed, ↓accuracy, ↑number of trials	
				19-Big object, square, rough, light ↑time, ↓speed, ↑accuracy, ↓numbers of trials	
			20-Big object, square, rough, light, ↓time, ↑speed, ↓accuracy, ↑number of trials	21-Small object, rectangular, rough, heavy, ↑time, ↓speed, ↑accuracy, ↓numbers of trials	
				23-Small object, square, rough, heavy, ↑time, ↓speed, ↑accuracy, ↓numbers of trials	
			22-Small object, rectangular, rough, heavy, ↓time, ↑speed, ↓accuracy, ↑number of trials	25-Small object, circular, rough, heavy, ↑time, ↓speed, ↑accuracy, ↓numbers of trials	
			24-Small object, square, rough, heavy, ↓time, ↑speed, ↓accuracy, ↑number of trials	27-Small object, rectangular, smooth, heavy, ↑time, ↓speed, ↑accuracy, ↓numbers of trials	
				28-Small object, rectangular, smooth, heavy, ↓time, ↑speed, ↓accuracy, ↑number of trials	

			26-Small object, circular, rough, heavy, ↓time, ↑speed, ↓accuracy, ↑number of trials 29-Small object, rectangular, rough, light ↑time, ↓speed, ↑accuracy, ↓numbers of trials 32-Small object, square, rough, light,↓time, ↑speed, ↓accuracy, ↑number of trials 35-Small object, square, smooth, light,↑time, ↓speed, ↑accuracy, ↓numbers of trials 37-Small object, circular, smooth, heavy,↑time, ↓speed, ↑accuracy, ↓numbers of trials	30-Small object, rectangular, rough, light, ↓time, ↑speed, ↓accuracy, ↑number of trials 31-Small object, square, rough, light ↑time, ↓speed, ↑accuracy, ↓numbers of trials 33-Small object, rectangular, smooth, light, ↑time, ↓speed, ↑accuracy, ↓numbers of trials 34-Small object, rectangular, smooth, light, ↓time, ↑speed, ↓accuracy, ↑number of trials 36-Small object, square, smooth, light, ↓time, ↑speed, ↓accuracy, ↑number of trials 38-Small object, circular, smooth, heavy, ↓time, ↑speed, ↓accuracy, ↑number of trials 39-Small object, circular, rough, light, ↑time, ↓speed, ↑accuracy, ↓numbers of trials 40-Small object, circular, rough, light, ↓time, ↑speed, ↓accuracy, ↑number of trials 41-Small object, circular, smooth, light ↑time, ↓speed, ↑accuracy, ↓numbers of trials 42-Small object, circular, smooth, light, ↓time, ↑speed, ↓accuracy, ↑number of trials.

Material used in Azzam reacquisition hand skill grading scale

1-Big object, rectangular shape, rough, heavy, ↑time, ↓speed, ↑accuracy, ↓numbers of trials

2-Big object, rectangular shape, rough, heavy, ↓time, ↑speed, ↓accuracy, ↑number of trials

3-Big object, square shape, rough, heavy, ↑time, ↓speed, ↑accuracy, ↓numbers of trials

4-Big object, square shape, rough, heavy, ↓time, ↑speed, ↓accuracy, ↑number of trials

5-Big object, rectangular, rough, light, ↑time, ↓speed, ↑accuracy, ↓numbers of trials

6-Big object, rectangular, rough, light, ↓time, ↑speed, ↓accuracy, ↑number of trials

7- Big object, rectangular, smooth, heavy, ↑time, ↓speed, ↑accuracy, ↓numbers of trials

8-Big object, rectangular, smooth, heavy, ↓time, ↑speed, ↓accuracy, ↑number of trials

9-Big object, circular, rough, heavy, ↑time, ↓speed, ↑accuracy, ↓numbers of trials

10-Big object, circular, rough, heavy, ↓time, ↑speed, ↓accuracy, ↑number of trials

11-Big object, rectangular, smooth, light, ↑time, ↓speed, ↑accuracy, ↓numbers of trials

12-Big object, rectangular, smooth, light, ↓time, ↑speed, ↓accuracy, ↑number of trials

13-Big object, circular, smooth, heavy, ↑time, ↓speed, ↑accuracy, ↓numbers of trials

14-Big object, circular, smooth, heavy, ↓time, ↑speed, ↓accuracy, ↑number of trials

15-Big object, circular, smooth, light, ↑time, ↓speed, ↑accuracy, ↓numbers of trials

16-Big object, circular, smooth, light, ↓time, ↑speed, ↓accuracy, ↑number of trials

17-Big object, rectangular, rough, light ↑time, ↓speed, ↑accuracy, ↓numbers of trials

18-Big object, rectangular, rough, light, ↓time, ↑speed, ↓accuracy, ↑number of trials

19-Big object, square, rough, light ↑time, ↓speed, ↑accuracy, ↓numbers of trials

20-Big object, square, rough, light, ↓time, ↑speed, ↓accuracy, ↑number of trials

21-Small object, rectangular, rough, heavy, ↑time, ↓speed, ↑accuracy, ↓numbers of trials

22-Small object, rectangular, rough, heavy, ↓time, ↑speed, ↓accuracy, ↑number of trials

23-Small object, square, rough, heavy, ↑time, ↓speed, ↑accuracy, ↓numbers of trials

24-Small object, square, rough, heavy, ↓time, ↑speed, ↓accuracy, ↑number of trials

25-Small object, circular, rough, heavy, ↑time, ↓speed, ↑accuracy, ↓numbers of trials

26-Small object, circular, rough, heavy, ↓time, ↑speed, ↓accuracy, ↑number of trials

27-Small object, rectangular, smooth, heavy, ↑time, ↓speed, ↑accuracy, ↓numbers of trials

28-Small object, rectangular, smooth, heavy, ↓time, ↑speed, ↓accuracy, ↑number of trials

29-Small object, rectangular, rough, light ↑time, ↓speed, ↑accuracy, ↓numbers of trials

30-Small object, rectangular, rough, light, ↓time, ↑speed, ↓accuracy, ↑number of trials

31-Small object, square, rough, light ↑time, ↓speed, ↑accuracy, ↓numbers of trials

32-Small object, square, rough, light, ↓time, ↑speed, ↓accuracy, ↑number of trials

33-Small object, rectangular, smooth, light, ↑time, ↓speed, ↑accuracy, ↓numbers of trials

34-Small object, rectangular, smooth, light, ↓time, ↑speed, ↓accuracy, ↑number of trials

35-Small object, square, smooth, light, ↑time, ↓speed, ↑accuracy, ↓numbers of trials

36-Small object, square, smooth, light, ↓time, ↑speed, ↓accuracy, ↑number of trials

37-Small object, circular, smooth, heavy, ↑time, ↓speed, ↑accuracy, ↓numbers of trials

38-Small object, circular, smooth, heavy, ↓time, ↑speed, ↓accuracy, ↑number of trials

39-Small object, circular, rough, light, ↑time, ↓speed, ↑accuracy, ↓numbers of trials

40-Small object, circular, rough, light, ↓time, ↑speed, ↓accuracy, ↑number of trials

41-Small object, circular, smooth, light ↑time, ↓speed, ↑accuracy, ↓numbers of trials

42-Small object, circular, smooth, light, ↓time, ↑speed, ↓accuracy, ↑number of trials

N.B, The time required to perform the level in normal from 180sec to 200 sec. We use the stop watch to measure the time performance the more decrease in time of performance indicate to improvement in gaining the skill

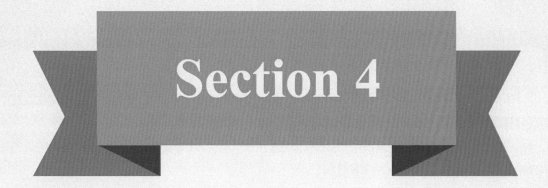

Section 4

Evaluation of fine motor skill

- Evaluation methods
- Skill analysis
- Standaradized tests for fine motor skills evaluation

Evaluation of fine motor skills

Upper extremity function plays an important role in gross motor skills such as crawling, walking, and the ability to recover balance and protect the body from injury, it become apparent that upper extremity function is the basis for fine motor skills as reaching, grasping and eye hand coordination .

Key element of fine motor skills:

1-Eye-hand co-ordination also called visual regard for locating a target

2-Reaching involving transportation of the arm and hand in space as well as postural support

3-Grasp including grip formation, grasp, and release

4-Hand manipulative skills

Neural components of fine motor skills:

1-Motor process including the co ordination of the eyes, head, trunk, and arm movement and co ordination of both the transport and grasp phases of reach.

2-Sensory process including the co ordination of visual, vestibular, and somato sensory system.

3-Internal representation important for the mapping of sensation to action.

4-Higher level processes essential for adaptive and anticipatory aspects of manipulatory function

Evaluation methods

a-History taking:

1-list any concern about your child motor skills, activity of daily living, behavior and play skills.

2-Development and family information.

b-Informal evaluation:

Visual: how your child processes what he sees

Auditory: how your child processes what he hears

Tactile: how your child processes what he touch

Vestibular: how your child processes himself in motion

Proprioceptive: how your child processes his actual movement

c-Formal evaluation:
1)-Muscle tone assessment
2)-Range of motion including scapula- thoracic articulation
3)-Test of tightness including spinal flexibility
4)-Functional muscle test
5)-Sensory test: touch, pain, thermal sensation, sense of position, sense of movement
6) - Evaluation of motor control:

A-Postural reaction
- Without righting reaction the patients will have difficulty in getting up from the floor, getting out of bed, sitting up and kneeling.
- Without equilibrium reaction the patients will have difficulty in maintaining and recovering of balance in all positions and ADL activities.
- Without protective reaction the patients suffering from repeated fallen, difficulty to bear weight on the affected side during normal ADL activities

B-Reflexes:

-Asymmetrical tonic neck reflex:
Interfere with the following fine motor activities
- Can not bring an object to the mouth
- Can not hold an object in both hands
- Can not grasp an object in front of the body while looking at
- Loss of eye hand co ordination
- Can not move both arms in midline.

-Symmetrical tonic neck reflex:
Tonic labyrinthine reflexes interfere with all functional activities

Ass. Prof. Dr. Ahmed M. Azzam

-Positive supporting reaction:

The patients will have difficulty in Getting up from, sitting in a chair, walking down steps, maintain balance in standing

-Grasp reflex:

The patients will have difficulty in all hand manipulative skills (grasping, reaching, eye hand co ordination)

7- Eye hand Co ordination tasks:

Bricks used to build a tower to test co ordination, writing, placing objects into containers, tossing and catching a ball,playing a board games and stacking cones are used to test co ordination.

8-Balance:

The ability to control the body position in space is essentials to moving one part of the body

Types of balance:

1-Static:

Maintain balance in static position as sitting and standing
- Evaluated by time by maintaining position in 30 sec.
     ex: -Double limb support
- Single limb support
- Heel-toe position(tandem)
- Romberg test

2-Dynamic:

Maintain balance when support surface move or when body move on stable surface.
objective test as biodex stability system

subjective by using:
- Rotatory chair, balance board, medical ball
- Stand up, walking, turning, stoop in and recovery

3-Automatic postural reaction:

as equilibrium and protective reaction maintain balance in unexpected external disturbance.

9-Grasping:

- Rattle demonstrate the ability to grasp and release in a very young child
- Bricks of varying size demonstrate ability to grasp, retain, and release,with the smaller ones posing relatively greater problems.
- Beads of varying size,being round, are harder to pickup and retain than bricks both bricks and beads can be put into container as a test of precision.
- Small sweets provide an incentive as well as demonstrating the ability to pic up a tiny objects and to retain grip while transferring to the mouth.
- Small pegs and a board are used to test fine grip and precision.
- Posting boxes and shape board give some evidence of ability to recognize shape as well as testing of manipulative skills. shape board should have three or four geometric shapes .A screw peg and nuts require a certain manipulation as well as testing of pronation and supination pencil and papers are used for testing dexterity, sustained control of a small object in use as well as copying ability.

Pencil should be of varying thicknesses to accommodate varying strengths of grip. Human grasping movements either power or precision grips which can be used alternatively or in combination for every type of object. precision grips used for writing and power grip for hammering

1-Use a power grasp on tool such as eating, tooth brush, hammer.
2-Modify use of a radial grasp according to pressure requirement for small objects.
3-Supinate the fore arm during grasp.
4-Use of full palmar grasp with wrist extension and varying degree of elbow flexion and extension

10-Voluntary release:

1-Release objects that are stabilized by supporting surface (as pegboard)

2-Voluntary release alight objects onto a flat surface

3-Place an object within 1 inch of the other objects without disturbed these by using finger extension

4-Release object while maintaining the fore arm in mid position

11- Hand manipulation:

1-Use shift skills in handling fastener son clothes

2-Use shift skills in managing paper for cutting

3-Use of translation and shift skills in handling money

4-Use pencil appropriately in hand

5-Use of simple rotation to open and close bottles

12-Bilateral skills:

1-Stabilize small containers by grasping with one hand while the other hand places objects into the containers

2-Stabilize paper effectively with one hand during a brief coloring activity

3-Manipulate paper by shifting with the non preferred hand while using scissors to cut with the other hand

13-Reaching:

Reaching for an object can be divided into two sub component reach and grasp which appear to be controlled by separate areas of the brain. Children with pyramidal lesion show a great problem with grasp component of reaching although transport component may be normal this suggest that extra pyramidal tract may control proximal muscles involved in reaching movement while pyramidal pathway are required for the fine motor control of grasping movement.

- In spastic patients the transport and grasp components will be affected the patient will recover the reach phase earlier and more completely than grasp phase, the two components require coordination to be functionally effective .The grasp part of reaching tested as before the transport part tested by bring two cups one large filled with water the other small empty then ask child to pouring water in empty cup and the opposite.

Two distinct and coordinated movement components included in reaching:

Transporting phase (extra- pyramidal control) which bring the hands to the target, in this part of movement mainly the proximal muscles and joints are involved, movement knowledge of the position of the object in the room is needed

Grasp phase (pyramidal control) in which the hand is shaped in anticipation of contact with the object this phase involve mainly the distal joints and muscles, perception of size and the shape of the object is needed.

Although the grasp and transport phase of reach are separately controlled they are coordinated so that the grasp phase starts during the transportation phase.

Functional problems have fine motor components:
Poor hand writing
Difficulty in managing materials in the class room
Difficulty with art work including scissor use
Limited constructive play skills
Avoidance of play with peers
Messy eating
Slow dressing with avoidance of fasteners
Lack of independence in getting ready for schools

Skill analysis

Four areas are analyzed:
1-Sensation:
Including the ability to detect changes in touch, visual and auditory stimuli
2-Motor skills:
Basic strength and flexibility, motor control, motor planning and accuracy, balance and fine motor coordination
3-Perception:
Design copying
4-Intellect:

Decision making, problem solving

Examples:
EX1: Reaching and eye hand coordination
Product name: block towering games

Description: one version has a tall tower of rectangular blocks, patients must remove one block at a time and carefully place it on the top of the tower without making any of the block fall, another version uses of asymmetric pieces for towering

Adaptations: symmetric game pieces are easier then asymmetric ones. To make the game more challenging, blocks can be numbered with a pen or marker then patient must remove or place a specifically numbered block on their turn

EX2: Grasp
Product name: pegboards

Description: pegs and pegboards can be found in a variety of shapes, sizes, weight, and materials. The grasp pattern for holding and placement is most affected by the size of the peg being used

Adaptations: hand positioning and grasp patterns used can be affected by the position of the child (prone, sitting, standing) as well as the boards (horizontal, angel, vertical) difficulty can be increased by using pieces that have more than one peg to be lined up with a hole for placement, using rubberized boards or pegs also increases difficulty by adding resistance when pegs are placed and removed

Standardized tests for fine motor skills evaluation:

1-Aptitude test and Copying designs
Test perception

2-Threading beads and grooved peg board test
Test delicate movement+ finger dexterity

3-Building towers test
Test eye hand co ordination +grasping

4- Manual dexterity and Throwing and catching ball tests
Test eye hand co- ordination

5-Purdue peg board, finger dexterity and Writing by pencil tests
Test finger dexterity

6-Pouring water from large to small and opposite test
Test transport phase of reaching

7-Peg domino and Place object in container test
Test voluntary release

8-Stalking cones test
Test eye hand co ordination

9-9 hole Peg board test
Test grasping

10-Geometrical 4 shape board test
Test grasping

11-Screw and nut test
Test supination

12-Voluntary release object test
Test voluntary release

13-Fasteners clothes test
Test hand manipulative skills

14-Hand dexterity and Cutting with scissors tests
Test bilateral hand use

15-Handling money test
Test hand manipulative skills

16-Open and close bottles test
Test hand manipulative skills

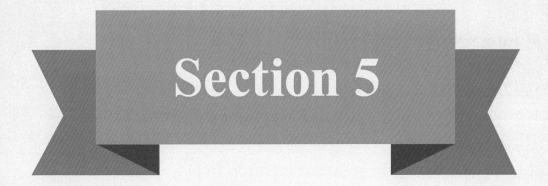

Section 5

Treatment of fine motor disorders

- Methods of treatment focus on fine motor problems
- Spasticity control
- Inhibition of released primitive reflexes
- Postural control
- Balance training is brain training
- Underlying mechanism of balance training
- Facilitation of delayed mile stone
- Traditional physiotherapy program
- Sensory integration therapy
- Sensory integration tools
- Specific treatment suggestions for enhancing supination
- General intervention principles for grasp problem
- Strategies used to enhance voluntary release
- General principles for developing hand manipulative skills
- Specific treatment of hand dysfunction in rehabilitation

Treatment of fine motor disorders:

Goals of intervention program:

1-Preventoin:
The potentials of primary or secondary problems is minimized
2-Modification:
The child changes based on self participation in activities
3-Remediation:
Facilities change to modify or enhance skills
4-Compensation:
Action or task is modified
5-Maintenance:
Ongoing use of the skills is encouraged

Methods of treatment focus on fine motor problems:

1-Positioning of the child and the therapist

2-Inhibition of tone and released abnormal pattern

3-Postural control (postural reaction training, facilitation of mile stone, traditional program)

4-Sensory integration approach

5-Isolated arm and hand movement

6-Grasp

7-Voluntary release

8-Hand manipulation

9-Bilateral skills

10- Integration of skills into functional activities

11-Reaching

12-Specific treatment of hand dysfunction in rehabilitation

(1) Positioning of the child and the therapist
The most commonly used position for treatment and functional use of fine motor skills is sitting. When table is used it should be at or very slightly above

elbow height. Using of lowering table facilitate upper trunk flexion, internal rotation of shoulder which limit of supination movement necessary for fine motor activities. Using of higher table facilitate abduction and internal rotation which hindering the supination movement

(2) Inhibition of tone and released abnormal pattern:

-Spasticity control
-Inhibition of primitive reflexes

Prolonged stretch to spastic muscle to gain relaxation via: At first quick stretch occur lead to stimulate gamma fibers lead to stimulate con-tractile part of intra-fusal muscle fiber lead to stimulate non contractile part which include stretch receptors sending afferent signals to PHC Then to AHC then to alpha motor neuron causing contraction of extra-fusal muscle fibers.

At second step just one contraction or repeated contraction occurred stimulate GTO sending 1b afferent to PHC then to 1b inter neuron which reverses the stimulated signals into inhibitory signals. Then inhibit AHC then inhibit alpha motor neuron then relaxate extra-fusal muscle fibers. Techniques used as prolonged stretch (positioning, night splint, reflex inhibiting pattern, Bobath technique)

In most cases the abnormal pattern is due to combined forces of shortening and spasticity of the involved muscles (long-standing uncontrolled spasticity results in shortening of the muscle fibers and muscle sheath).

So these combined pathological mechanism is in bad need for proper physiotherapy program (via eliminate hyperirritability of the spastic muscles) plus adjustable static and dynamic splint (decrease and release of muscle and sheath contracture, relaxation of spastic muscles, stimulate Proprioceptive and cutaneous receptors by creating a deep pressure effect on the skin, inhibitions of pathologic reflexes and create the support needed to stabilize the extremities). The decrease of spasticity and tightness also help in development of muscle balance.

Spasticity control

1-Ice application :

- Prolonged application on spastic muscles with looking at hyperemia every minute to avoid burn will produce inhibition of gamma fiber .
- Brief application on anti-spastic muscle will produce firing of gamma fibers of anti-spastic muscle which produce reciprocal inhibition of spastic muscles.

2-Vestibular stimulation:

Static(in linear acceleration) or dynamic(in angular movement) vestibular stimulation stimulate crista ampularis and endolymph of semicircular canal stimulate vestibuo-cochlear nerve lead to stimulate the vestibule-spinal tract which modulate firing of alpha motor neuron leading to modulation of stretch reflexes of muscles leading to generalized relaxation of spasticity.

3-Balance training:

Balance contain three receptors(vision, vestibular system and proprioceptors) all these receptors are including in balance training we can isolate the vision by covering the eyes and isolate proprioceptors by standing on disturbed board so the concentration will be on vestibular stimulation. Vestibular system cannot be isolated it must included in balance training. Balance contain three components (righting reaction, equilibrium reaction and protective reaction)

Table 6) Components of balance:

Characteristics of reactions	Righting reaction	Equilibrium reaction	Protective reaction
1-Stimulus	By tilting	By disturbance	By forced movment
2-Response	Righting of head and thorax(axial part)	Upper side has equilibrium reaction, lower side has protective reaction and righting reaction on axial part	Step forward or backward or sideway to maintain balance

3-COG(center of gravity)	Within B.O.S	Within B.O.S	Outside B.O.S
4-Base of support(B.O.S)	Big	Small	Very small
5-End result of training(function outcome)	sitting	Standing and walking	Prevention of repeated fallen

Inhibition of spasticity occurred via vestibular stimulation,propricptive stimulation and facilitation of postural reaction components which leasd to sensory information lead to sensory motor integration and end by motor strategy which mean gaining of function after decreasing of spasticity.

4-Faradic stimulation :

electric-stimulation of anti-spastic muscles produce depolarization of the skin and muscle produce contraction of anti-spastic muscle which stimulate the reciprocal inhibition mechanism by contraction of ant-spastic muscle and relaxation of spastic one.

5-Vibration:

- Vibration by high frequency on anti-spatic muscle lead to stimulation of Ia afferent leading to muscle activation and reciprocally relax the spastic one via reciprocal inhibition mechanism.
- Vibration by low frequency on spastic muscle lead to inhibition of Ia afferent due to adaptation leading to relaxation of spastic muscle

6-Approximation:

Static(weight bearing) and dynamic(manual approximation and walking) approximation stimulate the static and dynamic prpoprioceptors which transferred to dorsal colum tracts which localized by sensory area and smoothening by cerebellum and basal ganglion aiming for engramed to motor area and modulate the tone surrounding. Slow approximation used to inhibit spasticity.

7-Irradiation

Using resistance to strong muscle for firing of motor neuron pool of weak muscles.

8-Trigggering of mass flexion

Stimulate the flexion pattern in L.L produce inhibition of extensor spasticity via(clenching of toes, painful stimuli to sole of the foot,firm pressure to shaft of tibia and electric stimulation to anterior tibial group) produce mass flexion of LL leading to relaxation of extensor spasticity.

9-Positioning

- Quadruped position is recommended due to it has the following effects (prolonged stretch to flexors of upper limbs and extensors of lower limb-static approximation-inhibition of primitive reflexes –inhibition of released abnormal pattern). Produce reflex inhibiting pattern leading to relaxation of spastic muscles.

10-Prolonged stretch

Prolonged stretch to spastic muscle to gain relaxation via: At first quick stretch occur lead to stimulate gamma fibers lead to stimulate con-tactile part of intra-fusal muscle fiber lead to stimulate non contractile part which include stretch receptors sending afferent signals to PHC then to AHC then to alpha motor neuron causing contraction of extra-fusal muscle fibers. At second step just one contraction or repeated contraction occurred stimulate GTO sending 1b afferent to PHC then to 1b inter neuron which reverses the stimulated signals into inhibitory signals. Then inhibit AHC then inhibit alpha motor neuron then relaxate extra-fusal muscle fibers. Techniques used as prolonged stretch (positioning, night splint, reflex inhibiting pattern, Bobath technique)

11-Night splint

Produce prolonged stretch aiming for relaxation of spastic muscles and passive stretch for tight muscles

12-Casting

Produce prolonged stretch aiming for relaxation of spastic muscles and passive stretch for tight muscles

13-Biofeedback

Visual and auditory stimulation to anti-spastic muscles produce reciprocal inhibition of spastic muscles

14-Bobath technique

Depend on putting the spastic limb in (positioning, reflex inhibiting pattern, facilitation of postural reaction) using proximal and distal key point of control. Bobath technique leading to relaxation of spastic muscles via prolonged stretch

15-Topical anesthesia

- desensitization of the skin+ inhibition of gamma fiber of spastic muscles via spraying of anesthesia in one direction 3- 5 times then distribute it all over the spastic muscles cover it and leave for a minutes will produce relaxation.

16-Facilitate to anti-spastic muscle

Via tactile stimulation+ quick stretch +active contraction
Produce reciprocal inhibition to spastic muscles

17-Placing technique

Weight bearing to spastic limb on anti-spastic position produces prolonged stretch on spastic muscles and relaxation by putting upper limb in extension and lower in flexion and maintain position will produce relaxation.

18-Invertwd head position

one method of vestibular stimulation(lateral and antero-posterior swinging from upside-down (static vestibular stimulation) and rotatory movement from upside down(dynamic vestibular stimulation) produce generalized relaxation via stimulation of vestibu-lospinal tracts which modulate alpha motor neuron and in sequence modulate stretch reflex of spastic muscles.

19- Hot packs

Stimulate arterial receptors leading to vasodilatation and increase of elasticity of spastic muscles leading to decrease tension of extroceptors on spastic muscles.

20-Graduated active ex. for anti- spastic muscles

Starting with tapping followed by passive movement on anti-spastic muscles till the patient share in (active assisted) then active participation producing reciprocal inhibition to spastic muscles.

Inhibition of released primitive reflexes

1-Grasp reflex

The inhibition of the reflex can be achieved by:

A-Hand weight bearing from quadruped and side sitting position.

B-Reflex inhibiting pattern for U.L from sitting position as thumb extension pattern as distal key point of control.

C-Encourage hand function as reaching and voluntary release

2-Asymmetrical tonic neck reflex

To inhibit this reflex:

A-positioning:

- Encourage the child to assume side lying position

- Quadruped position

B-Reflex inhibiting pattern:

From sitting position (on roll, on lap) apply the following pattern using proximal key point of control:

- All outward rotation.

- Horizontal abduction.

- Extension diagonal.

- Elevation.

C-Break-down the pattern of reflex.
When child in supine lying position, the head rotated to one side, the therapist adducts the arm on the face side and extend the arm on the occipital side.

D-Approximation to the head and upper limb to normalize the muscle tone (slow, rhythmic)...

E-Facilitation of postural reactions

F-Encourage hand function.

3-Positive supporting reaction
This reflex can be inhibited by:
a-Approximation for L.L (slow, regular and rhythmic)
b-Positioning e.g. quadruped, sitting on roll and squatting.
c-Reflex inhibiting pattern.
-Dorsiflexion of toes and ankle as distal key point of control
-Flexion, abduction and external rotation as proximal key point of control
d-Facilitation of dorsiflexion by
-Tapping in the anterior tibial group
-Painful stimulus to sole of the foot
-Pressure on the medial tibial plateau or medial malleolus
E-Facilitation of rolling and walking

3) Postural control
- postural reaction training
- facilitation of mile stone
- traditional program

The labyrinth:
1-Bony
2-Membranous (auditory cochlea)(non-auditory vestibular system)

Vestibular apparatus:

1-Static labyrinth: composed from saccule and utricle (orientation of head in space, linear acceleration, righting reaction, orientation during swimming)

2-Semicircular canal: composed of crista ampularis (angular acceleration)

The benefits of balance training are to continually increase the patient awareness of balance threshold or limits of stability by creating controlled instability. The somato-sensory, visual, and vestibular systems interact and contribute to the maintenance of sitting balance. They are considered the key of postural control, as each system must be integrated to determine the body's center of gravity (COG). It receives this information from peripheral sources such as muscles, joint capsules and soft tissue receptors (called muscle spindles, ruffini endings and pacinian corpuscles). This system plays an important role in regulating sitting balance.

The information must be detected peripherally and transmitted centrally for processing. These impulses stimulate the child postural reflex mechanisms. It affects multiple systems such as the sensory, musculoskeletal, limbic, vestibular, and ocular systems simultaneously, leads to different therapeutic benefits that will be evidenced in behavioral patterns used in sitting balance Sitting balance is considered the bottleneck stage of development because it is the separation between primitive a pedal stage and postural reaction stage which its developed lead functionally to sitting, standing, walking, prevent fallen.

Postural control of the head, neck, and trunk is essential for normal functions of the sitting level. The spastic diplegic patient must have control of the head and trunk to manage shifting and bearing weight in sitting to free an extremity for function. The establishment of head, neck, and trunk control allows for dissociation of the shoulder and pelvic girdles from the trunk and dissociation of the extremities from the girdles.

__Balance training is brain training__

Essentially, when using balance or postural stabilizing exercises, an individual perform actually brain training, as it stimulates various centers in the brain. When incorporating balance exercises in a patient's program, musculoskeletal reaction is not only improved, but also brain to joint connections, therefore improving reactivity. Reactivity is key to preventing falls in sitting stage. Balance leads to proper recruitment of joint stabilizing muscles, and maintains proper axis of rotation of the joint.

This leads to accurate proprioceptive information from the somato -sensory system as the joint capsule, muscle, and ligament structures. With proper somatosensory input, balance will be improved. Additionally, poor posture, such as thoracic kyphosis, and forward head posture also reduces spinal rotation. Spinal rotation and three-dimensional freedom of movement is needed to correct an individual when balance reaction is called upon. Overall, to train balance, strive for proper alignment so the body learns how to move to good posture for its position of strength and reactivity, and not to one of compensation.

Righting reactions can be trained in antero-posterior and lateral direction, oblique and other directions. Righting reaction training started by facilitation of rolling in different position. Sitting on an unstable surface moving arms or legs to shift center of gravity – Sitting on unstable surface in combination with traditional lifting exercises .When your vestibular system senses that your body is not erect, it triggers the righting reflex by stimulating the vestibular system which stimulate vestibule-spinal tract which modulate the gamma fibers lead to modulate stretch reflex lead to modulate abnormal co-contraction and posture sway in sitting leading to improvement of core stability and sitting balance.

The vestibular organs provide sensory information about motion, and spatial orientation. The organs in each ear include the utricle, saccule, and three semicircular canals. The utricle and saccule detect gravity (vertical orientation) and linear movement. The semicircular canals detect rotational head movements and are located at right angles to each other. When these organs on both sides of the head are functioning properly, they send symmetrical signals to the brain that are integrated with other sensory and motors systems. If vestibular dysfunction occurs early in development, it slows the development of righting, equilibrium and protective reactions and motor-control tasks such as sitting unsupported, standing, and walking.

Stable vision is important for learning to read and write and for developing fine and gross motor control. If left untreated, a vestibular disorder can have adverse consequences for a range of functions as the child grows to adulthood. concentration on vestibular system training occurred by make the child blindfolded within the modified balance board which lead to isolate of proprioceptors and vision so pure vestibular stimulation occurred which lead to stimulation of vestibule-spinal tract which modulate the excitability of alpha-motor neuron of stretch reflex lead to modulation of muscle tone allowing the functional sitting to occur after repletion and massed practice.

Sensory information is regulated dynamically and modified by changes in environmental conditions .Despite the availability of multiple sources of sensory information, in a given situation, the central nervous system (CNS) gives priority to one system over another to control balance in the orthostatic position .Nondisabled adults tend to use somato-sensory information from their feet in contact with the surface while standing in a controlled environment with a firm base of support (BOS) .Under this condition, somato-sensory afferents account for 70 percent of the information required for postural control, while vestibular afferents account for 20 percent and visual input for 10 percent

Visual and vestibular inputs are likely to be more relevant sources of information when proprio-ceptive information is unreliable, for instance, during sway .The ability to choose and rely on the appropriate sensory input for each condition is called sensory reweighting When one is standing on an unstable surface, for instance, the CNS increases sensory weighting to vestibular and visual information and decreases the dependence on surface somato-sensory inputs for postural orientation. On the other hand, in darkness, balance control depends on somato-sensory and vestibular feed-back. The ability to analyze, compare, and select the pertinent sensory information to prevent falls can be impaired in hemiparetic stroke patients.

The key for gaining standing balance is the equilibrium reaction training(via disturbance in different position with decrease of the BOS with maintaining on COG within base of support the functional end result of practice and repeated training are standing and walking).

The key for prevent repeated falling is protective reaction training by training of hopping reaction +parachute reaction in addition to equilibrium reaction(via forced movement which move the COG out side BOS make great disturbance the functional end result of practice and repeated training is prevent repeated falling.

In patients with stroke, balance impairments and decreased foot proprioception are positively correlated .Abnormal interactions between the three sensory systems involved in balance(somatosensory, vestibular feedback and vision) could be the source of abnormal postural reactions .In situations of sensory conflict, a patient with stroke can inappropriately depend on one particular system over another .Laboratory measurements of sensory organization demonstrate that patients with chronic stroke perform worse in conditions of altered somatosensory information and visual deprivation or inaccurate visual input .Excessive reliance on visual input may be a learned compensatory response that occurs over time .Relying on a single system can lead to inappropriate adaptations and, hence, balance disturbances.

The components of the nervous system, which play a major role in the maintenance of static standing balance, must integrate information of proprio-ceptive, vestibular, and visual sources. Proprio-ceptive feedback mechanisms, serving to correct externally or internally induced errors in position, velocity, and force of movement, have been suggested as supporting the fundamental process of coordinated accurate movements These mechanisms are the main source of sensory information in normal people for balance maintenance when the feet were on a fixed surface Therefore, the nervous system may weight the importance of proprio-ceptive information for static standing balance more than information from visual and vestibular sources.

Underlying mechanism of balance training

Balance control requires the interaction of the nervous and musculoskeletal systems and contextual effects.

The nervous system provides the following:
1-Sensory processing: for perception of body orientation in space provided by visual, vestibular, and somato-sensory systems.

2-Sensori-motor integration: essential for linking sensation to motor responses (centrally programmed postural adjustments that precede voluntary movement).

3-Motor strategies: for planning, programming and executing balance response. Information from peripheral receptors including visual, vestibular, and somato-sensory (proprioceptive including conscial which are joint receptors, unconscial proprioceptors which are muscle spindle and GTO in addition to cutaneus receptors) to the cord and brain stem then be sensitized by the thalamus then localized by post central gyrus (sensory areas) to make three functions (perception of sensation, cognition, formation of sensory strategies) then reach to cerebellum and basal ganglion to prevent excessive activity, smoothening of information then to the pre-central gyrus which perform permanent changes lead to motor strategies and long term memory of this skill this means increase of anatomical (numbers) and physiological (efficiency) of synapses this means formation new neurological circuit which means learning of balance skill then formation of motor command via tracts to final common pathway (alpha and gamma MN) which provides two motor response

Enviromental factors affecting on balance:
- Closed or open environment.
- Surface(stable,unstable-firm, slippery-type of shoes)
- Amount of lighting

- Effect of gravity
- Well learned, new N.B; stable support surface primary maintained by somatosensory input
- Disturbed support surface vision become dominant
- vision and surface disturbance vestibular become dominant

Motor response to balance training

1) Internal:
- Reflex as stretch reflex
- Voluntary response
- Automatic postural response as equilibrium, protective reaction

2) External :
- Ankle strategies
- Weight shift strategies
- Hip strategies
- Stepping strategies

Facilitation of delayed mile stone

1-Facilitation of head control:

A-From prone:
- On roll and make bilateral elevation of shoulder
- On wedge tapping on forehead, painful stimuli on nose,
- On wedge make scapular retraction with paraspinal stimulation
- On wedge raising to on limb sudden drop then raising both limbs sudden drop
- On ball bounce the ball
- On ball facilitation of righting and equilibrium reaction, protective reaction

B-Supine:
- Pull to sit
- Pull to sit with painful stimuli on sternum
- Approximation must be slow in all cases

- Facilitation of postural reaction on ball

C-Sitting
- Approximation must be slow in all cases
- Bilateral extension diagonal
- Bilateral horizontal abduction
- Bilateral elevation without ward rotation

2-Facitition of rolling:

A-Blanket and two therapist raise the blanket from one side to initiate rolling
B-Sponge mattress pressure on it from one side
C-Counter rotation
- Shoulder against pelvis
Pelvis against shoulder
Shoulder, pelvis against each other

3-Facilitation of sitting:

A-Facilitation of trunk control by approximation of trunk on sitting
B-From supine to side sitting on wedge
C-Sitting on adjustable chair and support lower limb and foot on wedg
D-Sitting on chair and table in front of him to support him and lower it gradually when occur improvement in trunk control
E-Righting, equilibrium and protective reaction onball
F-Sitting on corner
G-Counter poisoning reaching while sitting
H- Static sitting with arm supported without arm supported from cross sitting long sitting, ring sitting

4-Facilitation of standing:

A-From supine to stand
B-From prone to quadruped to kneeling to haiif kneeling to standing by holding him from pelvis

C-Approximation of lower limbs

D-Standing frame

E-Manual standing by locking knee

F-Equilibrium reaction from standing

G-Standing with disturbance with holding a stand bar

H-Step forward and back ward with disturbance

I-Standing on one leg with disturbance

J-Standing on balance board

K-Standing on corner and disturbance

L-Stoop and recovery from flexion trunk and return, from squatting to standing

5-Facilitation of walking:

1-Closed environment

Between parallel bars hold him from axilla at shoulder level then make reciprocal movement

Using obstacles while I hold him like walking

2-Open environment

Gait training while child completely independent

Walk on wedge then between rolls as obstacles

Walk in one line, side way, one leg pass the other leg in side walking

Traditional physiotherapy program:

1-Training of pelvic stability and equal weight shift on both sides

2-Approximation technique for the upper and lower limbs

3-Training of active trunk extension for improving postural control and balance

4-Graduated active ex for trunk lower and upper limb muscles

5- Passive stretching ex. For tight muscles

6-Gait training ex

4) Sensory integration therapy

Sensory integration therapy, as practiced by the therapists, uses play activities in ways designed to change how the brain reacts to touch, sound, sight and movement. While the therapy is not new, it has remained somewhat controversial.

Sensory processing (sometimes called "sensory integration" or SI) is a term that refers to the way the nervous system receives messages from the senses and turns them into appropriate motor and behavioral responses. Whether you are biting into a hamburger, riding a bicycle, or reading a book, your successful completion of the activity requires processing sensation or "sensory integration.

The goal of sensory integrative therapy is to facilitate the development of the nervous system's ability to process sensory input in a more normal way. Sensory integration is a term for a process in the normal brain which pulls together all of the various sensory messages in order to form coherent information on which we can act. Basically everything we do requires sensory integration. This normal process can be missing or very badly organized in some people, notably autistic individuals.

The problem with sensory integration dysfunction children might be in the reticular formation. This area in the brain is responsible for keeping the brain alert and organized. Others has shown that the cerebellum is involved in sensory integration dysfunction children

There appear to be three major areas which are addressed with sensory integrative therapy

1- Vestibular 2- Proprioceptive 3-Tactile.

The vestibular system, located in the inner ear, relates us to gravity. It gives us our sensation of the weight of our body. It also tells us where we are in space, standing up, or on our head; whether we are falling, or turning our head. It monitors our head and body movements in any direction. It works 24 hours a day, and therefore is a very big source of input.

The proprioceptors are the neuro -receptors in tendons, muscles and joints. They tell us where our foot is when we pull it back to kick a ball, or how high our hand is when we reach up to comb our hair. Because the proprioceptors are getting input whenever we move, they also are a large source of sensory input. Proprioceptive input can vary in intensity. When one jumps on a trampoline, there is more intense input to the ankles, knees, and hips than there is in walking. Pushing a wheelbarrow full of cement is more intense input to the wrists, elbows and shoulders than pushing an empty wheelbarrow.

The tactile or touch system has three different types of receptors. One responds to light touch, like touching a hair on one's hand. This is a protective, alerting sense which makes us check on what is touching us in case it might be dangerous, like a bug crawling on the skin. The second receptor is for discriminative touch, for example when you reach in a pocket and know by feel whether you are touching your house key or your car key. We learn a great deal more than we generally realize through this sense of discriminative touch. The third set of touch receptors are those which receive information about heat, cold, and pain.

When a therapist offers sensory integration therapy, does it also involve other senses, such as smell, taste, vision and hearing. Sensory integration therapy works with all the senses, but the vestibular, tactile, and proprioceptive senses are important because they are such large sources of input. Of course, they are connected to everything else. For example, the vestibular system and the visual system are very closely associated, and often a child's ability to use his eyes in a coordinated way will improve as he/she receives enough vestibular input.

Hearing is also very important, of course, and one of the things that we offer is "auditory integration training" which aims to help balance the way the nervous system receives auditory input so that the child will not be hyper-responsive to particular sounds or to auditory input in general.

Sensory integration also uses therapies such as deep pressure, brushing, weighted vests, and swinging. Changing the foot surfaces and change the hand surfaces temperature, textures, pulling objects from sands and rice. These therapies appear to sometimes be able to calm an anxious child

<u>Sensory integration tools</u>

<u>1-Occupational therapy tactile discs</u>
<u>2-Pull and stretch bounce ball Colors may vary</u>
<u>3-Gymnic Disc and Sit Cushion</u>
<u>4-Feel and find</u>
<u>5-Dado square</u>
<u>6-Sensory shapes</u>
<u>7-Swings sensory tool</u>
<u>8-Dressings (buttons and ropes)</u>
<u>9-Teachable touchable : texture squares for matching and sorting</u>
<u>10-Gripables cutlery</u>
<u>11-Penagain</u>
<u>12-Pencil weight and pencil grip</u>
<u>13- Modified sponge, fork and scissor</u>
<u>14-Weighted(t-shirt-lap pad,blanket,vest)</u>
<u>15-Diving and playground dolphin</u>
<u>16-hand grip exercise</u>

<u>5) Isolated arm and hand movements</u>

Children find it easier to work on a movement component in isolation from other movement component Supination and pronation, wrist flexion and extension, M/PH joints flexion and extension with IP extension may be concentrated in skills training as tapping a table using the desired upper extremity motion. The therapist assist in isolation and stabilization by stabilize more proximal part e.g. stabilize the humerus if using supination and pronation, the forearm if using wrist flexion and extension,the dorsum of the hand if using MP flexion and extension .

Supination is a particularly difficult movement component for children with abnormal tone to use (hyper or hypo tonic patients stabilize in full pronation when doing fine motor task). Various degree of supination is critical for hand function Full pronation interferes significantly with thumb mobility and distal finger control The ability to use full supination is helpful in performing activities but for functional hand use the most important range of supination seems to be from full pronation to mid-position Use of supination is easiest when the humerus is adducted and elbow is flexed It is much more difficult to use supination when the humerus is in 90 degrees of flexion and the elbow is fully extended or the humerus is in full horizontal adduction and the elbow is extended.

In normal development babies work first on using supination when elbow in great deal of flexion, supination can be observed as babies brings their hands and toys to their mouths in supine,supported sitting,and prone on forearm.

Supination is a particularly difficult movement component for children with abnormal tone. Even children with only slightly low tone tend to stabilize in full pronation when engaging in fine motor tasks. Pronation

interfere significantly with thumb mobility and distal finger control being able to hold various degrees of supination is critical for higher levels hand skills, helpful in performing activities. The most important range of supination for functional skills use is between full pronation and mid-position.

During most skills that involve controlled use of the radial finger and thumb, the forearm is in approximately 30 to 45 degrees of supination12. The position from which the hand is able to function is when the forearm is midway between pronation and supination, the wrist in extension, the thumb in abduction and digits in moderate flexion in order for the hand to assume or maintain this functional position there need to be a balance between the extrinsic and intrinsic muscle groups of the forearm and hand, the wrist and digital joints.

Spasticity causes the rate of the affected muscle growth to be reduced causing disproportionate in muscles versus long bone growth. Consequently long bones grow at a faster rate than muscles as the muscle sarcomere are not arranged in the same longitudinal manner as

they are in normally innervated muscles. Thus muscle shortening occurs as a result of dynamic stretch reflex and reduced sarcomere formation lead to decrease of sarcomere numbers. The muscle that usually develops shortening first is pronator-teres muscle consequently supination of the forearm will be restricted.

By applying a low load prolonged stress to the shortened muscles at the end of their available range, they will ultimately be able to grow because the cross bridges between the myosine and actin filaments in the sarcomeres will be disrupted and peri-articular connective tissue stiffness will be reduced. When muscle is stretched on long run it responds by adding new sarcomere. This makes them return to their optimum tension generating length with no change to the muscle tendon.

Prolonged stretch is the key for decreasing of spasticity via stimulation of muscle spindle and golgi tendon organ. first step is firing of gamma fibers which connected with contractile part of intra-fusal muscle fiber producing contraction of contractile part and stretching of non contractile part of intra-fusal muscle fiber which stimulate stretch receptors(flower-spray, annulo-spiral receptors) sending impulses to Ia and II afferent to PHC to AHC to alpha motor neuron which produce contraction of extra-fusal muscle fiber lead to stimulation of golgi tendon organ which sending impulses to Ib afferent to PHC to Ib inter-neuron which reverse signals into inhibitory impulses which inhibit AHC which inhibit alpha motor neuron which inhibit extra-fusal muscle fiber produce relaxation of spastic muscles.

The passive stretch to contracted muscle and sheath which destruct adhesions in muscle and sheath increasing their elasticity and maintaining it. It has been appeared that most long standing pronation deformity are due to a combination of contracture of the involved muscles and their sheaths in addition to spasticity of the involved muscles. Tight pronator muscles cause an imbalance in forearm motor control which lead to poor hand functions and inability to perform ADL activity due to limited supination. The specialized treatment program produce improvement in all functional skills of the hand and dexterity of the fingers, which included the use of utensils for eating, improved handwriting skills.

Specific treatment suggestions for enhancing supination

1-Prolonged stretch to pronator teres, wrist flexors, elbow flexors to gain relaxation via Techniques used as prolonged stretch(positioning, night splint, reflex inhibiting pattern, Bobath technique).

2-Facilitation of anti-spastic muscles wrist extensors, elbow extensors, supinator: tapping followed by movement, quick stretch, triggering mass flexion, biofeedback, weight bearing, clenching to toes, compression on bony prominence, rapping the muscle, approximation, vibration, irradiation to weak muscles by strong muscles, ice application for brief time.

3-Passive stretching to tight muscles (pronators, wrist flexors, elbow flexors, shoulder adductor) to destruct adhesions in muscles and sheath. It must be decent gentle gradual stretch not over stretch at all ., lasting 20 second then relaxation 20 second 3-5 times per session then maintain the new range by using adjustable wrist splint plus supinator strasp after session for two hours then release for using the hand in ADL activity.

4-Graduated active exercise for upper limb muscles.

5- Gait training using aids in closed environment using obstacles, side walking then by pass walking to stimulate protective reaction for the hand

6-Hot packs to improve circulation and relax muscle tension applied on the forearm

7- Balance training program which include static and dynamic training

8-Encourage mouthing and finger feeding

9-Facilitate supination with the forearm on a surface as in weight bearing on floor, or on mat,while seated at a table the therapist place an object in the child hand,the child attempt to compensate for difficulty with supination by using wrist extension

10- Encourage the use of 45 to 90 degrees of supination followed by grasp of an object with elbow in 90 degrees of flexion,the child encourage to keep thumb up as reaching and grasping large birthday candles then put them into cake that require supination

11- Encourage lateral reach followed by grasp most of children with limited use of supination find it easier to combine humeral abduction with external rotation and supination than to use humeral flexion with external rotation and supination. Object presented laterally to the child allow the child to use abduction and external rotation which allow for supination

12-Encourage reaching by using shoulder flexion and external rotation by placing the object between leg and shoulder in sitting position depending on the child ability to control external rotation and supination while completing the reach

13-Encourage reaching across midline following stratigies suggested for reaching in front of the shoulder

14-Supination Ideas (Turning the hand over, palm up)Children were ringing water out of a towel by twisting it, turning pages of a book. "Guess which hand" games, where something is hidden in one hand, the partner guesses which by tapping the guest hand, A simple slinky is a great toy to encourage supination, Build with cones, grasping a magnet (adapt type and size to the child's needs),The The path is held with the non-affected hand and the child holds the magnet in the affected hand, under the path to guide the car.

15- Thumb abduction supination splint: it is supplied in rolls of various lengths and widths the 5 cm width roll was used for construction of the supination splints byplacing the loop of the roll through the child thumb then on a dorsum of the hand so it comes out on the ulnar side to volar part then dorsal again, overlap the part around the wrist, then continually up to forearm then around the elbow to epicondyles

6) Grasp

Therapist determine if grasp pattern is possible for the child or not according to the size of the objects with which it can be used that is larger ones, medium, small and tiny object.

Some children can use grasp pattern on larger object but not on small and tiny object due to lesser degree of stability

Children with poor stability in their hands tend to use a palmar grasp on tools as knives, toothbrushes, hairbrushes, and hammers rather than a power grasp in which the ulnar fingers provide stability for the handle and the radial finger are more extended

General intervention principles for grasp problem

1-If fisted hand is a problem concentrate on voluntary hand opening
Upper extremity weight bearing used to facilitate finger extension with finger extension
Stretching for finger and wrist flexors to facilitate grasping
Weight bearing splint
Tactile and proprioceptive input

2-Address supination and wrist stability
wrist stability may be addressed through use of hand weight bearing
wrist extension used more with small diameter objects in some children wheres others used more with larger diameter

3-Considering the stability of the child

Babies who were beginning to develop control of particular grasp pattern were most successful when grasping from a very firm surface and less successful on unstable surface

4-Consider object characteristics and orientation of object

The size, shape, weight, texture, and slipperiness of the objects must be given careful consideration Children can handle blocks and other objects with straight sides more effectively than round objects

Grasp of small tiny object should not be the priority for children, people use an opposed pattern to grasp items as a cup (cylinderic grasp,a ball (aspheric grasp),a telephone receiver and a large block

Children with disability be assisted in developing skills of all types of opposed grasp pattern, power grasp, and lateral pinch

5-Consider grasp without reach

To reach and grasp the child is required to preposition the arm and hand often against gravity

In treatment of grasp children respond better to intervention in which they only have to preposition the hand.

Levels of grasp training

Level 1grasp from therapist finger:

The child is in sitting position with shoulder adducted and forearm stabilize on his leg or table surface the therapist place the object at the child fingers the therapist note the degree and quality of wrist extension and finger and thumb position in the grasp

Level 2 grasp from palm of therapist hand:

The position as before but the therapist place object in the palm of his hand with hand sufficiently cupped to stabilize object,therapist place his hand under the child hand

Level 3 grasp from surface:

Now the object is placed on the table surface, therapist may find it helpful to place the object on a non skid surface or to stabilize the object with finger

Level 4 grasp from surface further from body with object in front of shoulder

At this level the child begin to combine supported reaching with preparation of the hand for grasp

Level 5 grasp from surface near midline

The child now begin to work on grasping at midline while controlling the hand, forearm, and elbow position

Level 6 grasp with object off surface

At this level the child needs to control the shoulder against gravity and control the degree of external rotation used.

7) Voluntary release

Motor control problems with voluntary release result from three key areas of difficulty:

1-poor arm stability 2-increased flexor tone 3-lack of effective use of intrinsic muscles of the hand

Problems are seen in poor IP joint extension or poor MP joint control. A typical pattern seen in poor quality voluntary release is MP joint extension with or without IP joint extension. Lack of extensor activity appropriately balanced with flexor activity interferes with effectiveness and efficiency of voluntary release. Some children with these problems resort to using tenodesis action by flexing at the wrist to initiate the voluntary release and may use the same pattern to initiate grasp.

Strategies used to enhance voluntary release

1-Hand weight bearing help the child to develop improved co contraction at the scapulo- humeral area, the elbow, and the wrist.

2-Reaching activities that involve touching a desired target and holding that position for a few second be helpful

3- Teaching the child to stabilize the arm against the body or on a surface prior to opening the hand be helpful compensatory strategies

4-Facilitation of supination, abduction and external rotation make it easier for the child to use elbow extension and supination which allow for voluntary release with wrist extension

5- Releasing into the container placed on the floor or at lower than the seat of the child chair learn the child to relax finger flexors

6-As children develop more control with voluntary release therapist can gradually decrease object, weight, stability, and size of the area used for object placement

8) Hand manipulation

There are five basic types of hand manipulation skills:

1-Finger to palm translation: movement of object from the finger to the palm

2-Palm to finger translation: movement of an object from the palm to the finger pads

3-Shift: slight adjustment of the object on or by the finger pads

4-Simple rotation: turning or rolling the objects 90 with the fingers acting as a unit

5-Complex rotation: turning an object over using isolated finger and thumb movement

Hand manipulation skills to be more effective the child should use some degree of supination and thumb opposition

General principles for developing hand manipulative skills:

1-Provide somato-sensory stimuli:
Many children with fine motor problems have difficulty with tactile perception.

Typical activities used for sensory awareness may include:

- Finding objects in beans, rice, or sand (graded finger movements are used to get the grains of rice or sand off the object),
- Pulling pieces of clay off a ball of a clay
- Pushing fingers into therapy putty or clay
- Stretching rubber bands around fingers

2-Facilitate the use of intrinsic muscles in grasp and hand functions:
- Pulling clay to facilitate use of intrinsic muscles
- Facilitate the use of MP flexion with IP extension due to this pattern require use of intrinsic muscles, and this is often the ending pattern after the child has complete the manipulation
- Emphasis on spherical grasp that use a combination of long flexor activity and intrinsic activity

3-Encourage use of bilateral manipulation:
- Infants manipulate objects between two hands
- Use of a surface on which to turn a puzzle piece and turning it within the hand

9) Bilateral hand use

In normal development babies develop gross symmetric bilateral skills such as (holding object with two hands, clapping, banging objects together)
Then stabilize objects with one hand while the other is manipulating (holding paper while coloring, holding a container while putting objects in)
Then manipulate objects with both hands simultaneously (stringing beads, tying a knot)
- The child may hold his hand on the paper while therapist draw a picture and ask child to guess what is being drawn.
Gradually the child is asked to do more with manipulated hand while using the stabilizing hand to maintain materials on the surface or in the grasp
- Padlock that key can be put into
- Markers with caps to put on
- A box with a lid and objects to put inside the box
- Hold a cup with one hand while putting object in with other hand

- Buttoning with both hands
- Tying a bow and doing craft project
- Fit blocks together

10) Integration of skills into functional activities

Integrating new skills into functional performance requires the involvement of parents or caretakers and teachers

11) Reaching

1-By using water mat game,have sponged objects floating within, encourage reaching and touching to make the object move
2-Busy boxes and rattles attached to playpen some of them are secured with tabletop with suction cup reaching is rewarded with sound movement
3-All exercises for grasping used for reaching Pediatric Occupational Therapists and Pediatric Physical Therapists

12) Specific treatment of hand dysfunction in rehabilitation

1-Reciprocate stimulation and antagonist used when there is paralysis of both agonist and antagonist.
2-Mesh gloves sensory stimulation
3-Mechanical hand arches training
4-Hand weight bearing (static and dynamic)
5-Spasticity control of hand muscles
6-Mirror therapy
7-Facilitatory techniques for LMN hand dysfunction
8-Sensory motor integration therapy for the hand(extroceptors, proprioceptors and vestibular training)
9-Bobath technique (extension-abduction) of the thumb based on prolonged stretch mechanism
10-Vestibular stimulation

11-Stimulate open active enriched environment via upsee therapy

12-Enhanced of forearm supination

13- Strengthing ex. of intrinsic and long flexors and extensors muscles

14-Night splint and dynamic splint

15-Positioning as placing technique and cat position

16-Facilitation of hand transfer from fingers to palm and opposite

17-ADL activities training

18-The best position for hand rehabilitation sitting position at the level of elbow or slightly above

19-Constrained bimanual therapy

20-PNF for hand muscles

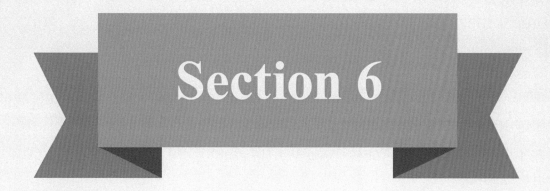

Section 6

References (for further reading)

1-Guo CB, Zhang W, Ma DQ, Zhang KH, Huang JQ (1996) Hand grip strength: an indicator of nutritional state and the mix of postoperative complications in patients with oral and maxillofacial cancers. Br J Oral Maxillofacial Surg 34: 325-327.

2-Ivanhoe CB, Reistetter TA (2004) Spasticity: the misunderstood part of the upper motor neuron syndrome. Am J Phys Med Rehabil 83: S3-S9.

3-van Meeteren J, van Rijn RM, Selles RW, Roebroeck ME, Stam HJ (2007) Grip strength parameters and functional activities in young adults with unilateral cerebral palsy compared with healthy subjects. J Rehabil Med 39: 598-604.

4-Rose VD, Shah SY (1987) A comparative study on the immediate effects of hand orthoses on reduction of hypertonus. J Aust Occup Ther 34: 59-64.

5-Frederiksen H, Gaist D, Petersen HC, Hjelmborg J, McGue M, et al. (2002) Hand grip strength: a phenotype suitable for identifying genetic variants affecting mid- and late-life physical functioning. Genet Epidemiol 23: 110-122.

6-Backman CA, Gibson GF, Parsons JR. Assessment of hand function: The relationship between pegboard dexterity and applied dexterity. Canadian Journal of Occupational Therap. 1992; 59(4): 208–213.

7-Chan TH, Forssberg H. An investigation of finger and manual dexterity. Perceptual and MotorSkills. Developmental Medicine and Child Neurology .2002;90(6): 537–542.

8-Eliasson AC, Burtner PA. The evidence-base for upper extremity intervention for children with cerebral palsy. In Improving hand function in children with cerebral palsy: Theory, evidence and intervention.; Journal of Pediatrics. 2008;67(8):231-236

9-EliassonAC, Krumlinde LU, Shaw K E,Wang CY .Effects of constraint-induced movement therapy in young children with hemiplegic cerebral palsy. Developmental Medicine and Child Neurology.2010; 47(4):266-275.

10-Exner C E,Lieber RL. In-hand manipulation skills in normal young children: A pilot study. OT Practice.2009; 56(7): 63– 72.

11-Graham K, Shaw K E. Botulinum toxin-A in cerebral palsy: functional outcomes. Journal of Pediatrics, 2000; 137(3):300-303.

12- Hoare BJ, Russo RO. Upper-limb movement training in children following injection of botulinum neurotoxin A. In International Handbook of Occupational Therapy Interventions Edited by Springer Publishers2009;P:343-350.

13-Hoare BJ, Wallen MA, Imms C, etal. toxin A as an adjunct to treatment in the management of the upper limb in children with spastic cerebral palsy. Developmental Medicine and Child Neurology.2010;52(9):543-550.

14-Hoare BJ, Imms CG, Carey LJ,Wasiak J K. Constraintinduced movement therapy in the treatment of the upper limb in children with hemiplegiccerebral palsy: a Cochrane systematic review. Clinical Rehabilitation,2008; 21(8):675- 685.

15- Kuhtz PH, Krumlinde LU, Eliasson CO ForssbergGH. Quantitative assessment of mirror movements in children and adolescents with hemiplegic cerebral palsy. Developmental Medicineand Child Neurology. 2000;42(6):728-736.

16-Carey L.M. : Somato-sensory loss after stroke. Critical Reviews in Physical Medicine and Rehabilitation Medicine 1995; 7: 51-91.

17- George H. K, Sally S. F and Margaret C. H:Techniques to improve arm and hand functionin chronic hemiplegia. Archives of Physical Medicine and Rehabilitation March 1992; 73: 220-227.

18-Humphrey D. R. and Freund H.J. Motor Control Concepts and Issues. New York, John Wiley & Sons, 1991.

19-kraft GH, Fitts SS and Hammond MC. Techniques to improve function of the arm and hand in hemiplegia. Arch Phys Med Rehab 2002; 73: 220-227.

20- Porter R.H and Lemon R.G: Cortico-spinal Function and Voluntary Movement . New York, sOxford University Press, 1995; 16(6): 34-40.

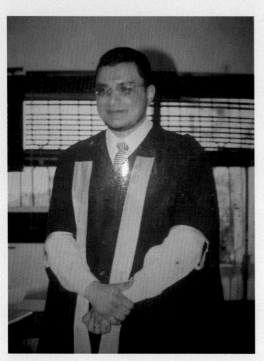

Dr.Ahmed Mohamed Azzam is an Egyptian assistant professor in pediatric rehabilitation from Mansoura city in the heart of the Niles Delta . Currently, he become ass. professor in Department of physiotherapy for developmental disturbance and pediatric surgery, Faculty of physical therapy, Cairo university, Egypt. Dr. Azzam has been awarded his PH.D degree in pediatric rehabilitation in Faculty of physical therapy, Cairo university, Egypt .He is holding a master degree in pediatric rehabilitation from Faculty of physical therapy, Cairo university, Egypt.

After 10 years of hard work, he finally issued his series of rehabilitation (essential mechanisms of neurological pediatric rehabilitation, essential mechanisms of orthopedic pediatric rehabilitation and Azzam scale in practical guide of occupational therapy). Dr. Azzam aimed at making pediatric rehabilitation interesting and of direct application to physiotherapy and occupational therapy .In our books text is linked with graphs, tables and diagrams to enable physiotherapy, occupational therapy students and readers to grasp real mechanisms that is essential for safe pediatric rehabilitation practice. Dr.Azzam sincerely hope that your reading of pediatric rehabilitation and occupational therapy books not only profitable to you but also stimulate your permenant interest in the fascinating subject of physiotherapy.

Printed in the United States
By Bookmasters